Smoothie for Healthy Sexual Health

The Complete Solution for Boosting Libido, Body Cleansing and Happy Life

Linda Pierce

Table of Contents

SMOOTHIE FOR HEALTHY SEXUAL HEALTH I

INTRODUCTION 7

CHAPTER 1 9

   SMOOTHIES RECIPES AND PREPARATION FOR INCREASED LIBIDO 9
      Beetroots Smoothie 9
      Pomegranate Smoothie 10
      Goji Berry or Wolf Berry Smoothie 11
      Maca or Peruvian Ginseng 13
      Bananas Smoothie 14
      Celery Smoothie 15

CHAPTER 2 16

   RECIPES AND PREPARATION FOR INCREASED SEXUAL DRIVE 16
      Avocado Smoothies 16
      Watermelon Smoothies 17
      Pumpkins Seed Smoothies 18
      Carrots Smoothie 19
      Banana Booster 20
      Chocolate Peanut Butter Smoothie 21
      Strawberry Stress Buster 22
      Chocolate Strawberry Banana Smoothie 23

CHAPTER 3 24

   FOODS THAT ENHANCES SEXUAL DRIVE 24
      Chili Peppers 24
      Avocado 24
      Raw Chocolate 25

    Bananas *26*
    Honey *26*
    Watermelon *27*
    Pine Nuts *27*
    Arugula *27*
    Figs *28*
    Strawberries *28*
    Pomegranates *28*
    Maca *29*
    Cinnamon *29*
    Ashwagandha *30*
    Coconut Oil *30*
    Almonds *30*

CHAPTER 4 .... **32**
    HOW TO IMPROVE YOUR SEX LIFE 32
    NUTRITIONAL TIPS FOR BOOSTING LIBIDO 33
        Ditch Endocrine-Disrupting Plastics *33*
        Don't Drink Plain Tap Water - Avoid Fluoride and Chlorine *34*
        Don't Eat Soy! *34*
        Quit Using Chemical-based Skin Products *35*
    THE TYPES OF FOODS TO EAT FOR AN IMPROVED SEX LIFE 35
        Eat Whole-Food Plants *35*
        Eat Foods Containing Zinc *38*
    REVIEW THE DRUGS YOU TAKE 38
    EMBRACE CHANGE OF TIME 39
    CONSULT BIOIDENTICAL HORMONE SPECIALIST 40

CHAPTER 5 .... **42**
    FOODS TO STAY AWAY FROM 42
        Sugar *42*
        Trans-Fats *42*
        Canned Foods *42*

    Soy *43*
    Salt *43*
    Alcohol *43*

CHAPTER 6 ....**44**

  UNDERSTANDING WOMEN EROGENOUS ZONES.. 44
    The Vulva *45*
    The G Spot *48*
  ORGASMS 49
    What physical adjustments happen within you during an orgasm? *51*
  HORMONE CHANGES DURING ORGASM 56
  SUPPORT FOR ORGASMS 59
  SEXUAL DESIRE 61

CHAPTER 7 ....**63**

  SOURCES OF POOR LIBIDO IN WOMEN 63
    Menopause *64*
    Progesterone deficiency *66*
    Polycystic ovarian syndrome *72*
    Fatigue *72*
    Stress *73*
    Depression *73*
    The oral contraceptive pill *75*
    Medications that reduce libido *78*
    Vaginal odor and infection *80*
    Herpes *82*
    Vaginismus *84*
    Pain in the region of the vulva *86*
    Urinary tract infections *89*
    Prolapse from the pelvic floor and/or vagina *90*
    Constipation *91*
    Poor blood circulation for the vulva *92*

CHAPTER 8 93

TREATMENT OPTIONS FOR LOW LIBIDO 93
- *Progesterone therapy* 93
- *Estrogen therapy* 103
- *Testosterone therapy* 109

CHAPTER 9 123

ENHANCING SEXUAL DRIVE IN MEN 123
- *Muscle Mass Building and Testosterone Enhancing* 123

WHAT TO EAT 125
- *Bacon Burgers.* 125
- *Chocolate Peanut Butter Shake.* 125
- *Nut-Crusted Salmon.* 125
- *Short Ribs.* 126
- *Grilled Salmon.* 126
- *No-Bun Burgers.* 126
- *Roasted Chicken.* 127
- *Slow-Cooker Stew.* 127
- *Steak and Eggs.* 127

CHAPTER 10 128

HERBS FOR BETTER SEX 128
- *Ginseng, "The King of Most Herbs"* 128
- *He Shou Wu- Fo-Ti, "Youthful Tonic"* 130
- *Ashwagandha, "Indian Ginseng"* 132
- *Guarana, "Sexier when Compared to a Cup of Joe"* 133
- *Creatine, "Muscle Powder"* 135
- *Astragalus, "The Fantastic Body Lifter"* 137

Copyright © 2021 by Linda Pierce

All rights reserved. No part of this publication may be reproduced, distributed, or transmitted in any form or by any means, including photocopying, recording, or other electronic or mechanical methods, without the prior written permission of the publisher, except in the case of brief quotations embodied in critical reviews and certain other non-commercial uses permitted by copyright law.

Introduction

Sex is among the greatest pleasures on the planet, since it serves a number of purposes, from relaxation to pleasure and sometimes manipulation. In whatever case it might be, we all come with an inbuilt desire to provide our partners the sexual satisfaction they crave, therefore the art of sex itself will not become an ordeal; a required evil.

Sadly, many couples are losing the sexual spark they once shared inside the bedroom, to an array of reasons which dwindling libidos worsened by unhealthy lifestyle choices is defined as the major culprit.

Dwindling libidos *is actually a resultant after-effect of financial pressures, stress at work, insufficient enthusiasm, monotony, unhealthy lifestyle and diet plan, etc.* Whatever the reason, there's a way to really get your groove again and satisfy your companion naturally without heavy reliance on performance enhancement drugs like viagra.

This is actually the purpose of this book. We will look into some typically common natural fruit and vegetable drink recipes, smoothies that boost sexual drive and libido in men and women.

Let's begin.

Chapter 1

Smoothies Recipes and Preparation for Increased Libido

Beetroots Smoothie

Beets continues to be used for years and praised as the best food for men, and it is abundant with *vitamin C and essential minerals like manganese and potassium.*

Frequent consumption of beetroots has immense benefits for health generally and libido specifically because they are highly concentrated with nitrates that get divided into nitric oxide. *Nitric oxide* generated by beetroots supports blood flow towards the penis, producing a stronger, fuller and sustained erection; giving the person a viagra-like effect, without medical effects of Viagra.

Ingredients

- ✓ Mid-sized Beetroot
- ✓ 3 bits of Celery Stalks
- ✓ 1 medium Lemon juiced
- ✓ 20 grams of ginger
- ✓ 1 medium apple

- ✓ 1 cup of clean water

Directions

- ✓ Wash all of your vegetables with clean water and one tablespoon of vinegar
- ✓ Cut them into small pieces prepared to be blended
- ✓ Pour in a blender
- ✓ Blend until smooth
- ✓ Pour in a glass and add ice
- ✓ And Voila! your juice is set to be consumed.

Pomegranate Smoothie

Pomegranate-Juice-Nutrition-and-Benefits

Pomegranates contain powerful anti-oxidants and were first regarded as the *symbol of fertility*. According to Researchers from your Queen Margaret University, One glass of pomegranate increases testosterone levels, acting as an all-natural aphrodisiac.

The analysis also proves they contain certain compounds comparable to sex steroids found within humans; this explains the partnership between pomegranates and increased sexual stamina and desires

Ingredients

- ✓ 1 cup of seeded pomegranates.
- ✓ 20 grams of ginger.
- ✓ 1 medium Lemon (juiced).

Directions

- ✓ Pour the seeded pomegranates inside a blender.
- ✓ Bring your peeled and cut ginger.
- ✓ Add the juiced lemon and a cup of water.
- ✓ Blend the mixture until very smooth.
- ✓ Pour out into a glass and then add ice.
- ✓ Your smoothie is set to be consumed.

Goji Berry or Wolf Berry Smoothie

Wolf Berry Juice

These berries are native to Asia and also have high anti-oxidant properties. It's mostly prepared like a sexual tonic to *boost sexual drive and stamina*. Consumption of Goji berries has been thought to increase testosterone levels, Improve sexual abilities, increase sperm quality and movement. Researchers have suggested increased consumption of Goji as a wholesome alternative to prescription of medications for erectile dysfunctions like Viagra.

Ingredients

- ✓ 1 peeled Banana
- ✓ ½ cup of dried Goji berries (soaked for a handful of hours)
- ✓ 10 grams of ginger
- ✓ 1 cup of Almond milk

Directions

- ✓ Pour the diced into the blender
- ✓ Supply your softened goji berries
- ✓ Put your diced ginger and almond milk
- ✓ Blend until mixture is smooth
- ✓ Pour in a glass and Serve with Ice.

The libido-enhancing smoothie becomes set to be enjoyed together with your lover.

Maca or Peruvian Ginseng

Maca or Peruvian Ginseng

This super fruit is native to the southern American and considered an *adaptogen,* at the top of the set of its immense benefits is increased testosterone as well as the tremendous boost it offers sex and fertility. *Increased intake of the black maca shows improved sperm production.*

Ingredients

- ✓ 1 tablespoon of dried maca powder.
- ✓ 1 cup of frozen Bananas.
- ✓ 1 or ½ cup of yoghurt or Almond milk.

Directions

- ✓ Pour your frozen bananas inside a blender.
- ✓ Add your yoghurt or almond milk to it.
- ✓ Then put a tablespoon of maca powder to the mixture.
- ✓ Blend until the mixture is smooth.
- ✓ Pour in a glass as well as your smoothie is ready.

Bananas Smoothie

Banana Smoothie and drink

Bananas are abundant with *potassium, magnesium, vitamin B1, vitamin A, Vitamin C, and Protein*; which are necessary for the improvement and production of sperms. In addition, it contains Bromelain, an enzyme in charge of increased libido and reversal of impotence in men.

Ingredients

- ✓ 2 mid-sized bananas peeled
- ✓ 10 grams of ginger
- ✓ 1 cup of Almond milk
- ✓ ½ cup of washed celery leaves

Directions

- ✓ Pour your diced bananas within a blender
- ✓ Add the celery leaves as well as your grated ginger
- ✓ Supply your almond milk to the mix
- ✓ And blend before the mixture is usually smooth
- ✓ Pour in a glass and then add ice as well as your smoothie is ready.

Celery Smoothie

Celery-smoothie and drink

They may be laced with *vitamin E, niacin, potassium, and magnesium*. In addition, it contains arginine, an amino acid which performs the same work as a sex enhancement by aiding the expanding of arteries.

Ingredients

- ✓ 2 cups of celery leaves
- ✓ 1 green apple (diced)
- ✓ 1 lemon(juiced)
- ✓ Almond or unsweetened yoghurt

Directions

- ✓ Pour your properly washed celery into a blender
- ✓ Put your apples and juiced lemon
- ✓ Add your almond milk or yoghurt
- ✓ Blend until smooth
- ✓ Pour in a cup then add ice and it is done to be consumed

Chapter 2

Recipes and Preparation for increased Sexual drive

Avocado Smoothies

<u>Avocado-Smoothie-Recipe</u>

They are saturated in folic acids, and so are an excellent source of vigor boost needed to keep things raunchy inside the bedroom. In addition, they contain healthy fats, Vitamin B and potassium; which function as a booster of male hormones necessary for virility in the bedroom.

<u>*Ingredients*</u>

- ✓ 2 large balls of avocado pears (seeds removed)
- ✓ ½ cup of frozen pineapples
- ✓ 1 cup of Almond milk
- ✓ 10 grams of ginger

<u>*Directions*</u>

- ✓ Place the seeded avocado within the blender
- ✓ Contribute the frozen pineapples
- ✓ Supply the ginger plus the Almond milk

- ✓ Blend everything together until smooth
- ✓ Pour in a glass and then add ice.

Watermelon Smoothies

Watermelon-Smoothie

This scarlet beauty is packed with Citrulline which aids the relaxation and dilation of arteries. Just about performing exactly the same functions as prescription medications targeted at treating erectile dysfunctions.

Ingredients

- ✓ 1 cup of watermelon with the seeds
- ✓ 1 little bit of apple (diced)
- ✓ 10 grams of ginger
- ✓ 1 cup of Almond milk or unsweetened yoghurt.

Directions

- ✓ Pour watermelon into the blender
- ✓ Put your apple and grated ginger
- ✓ Bring your milk or Yoghurt
- ✓ Blend everything together until smooth

- ✓ Pour right into a glass and serve with ice
- ✓ Pumpkins Seed Smoothies

Pumpkins Seed Smoothies

These are heavily packed with *potassium, niacin, calcium, phosphorus, and zinc,* which really is a prerequisite for the production of healthy sperms while boosting testosterone levels. Also, they are heavily packed with libido enhancing vitamins like *Vitamin B, C, K, D, E.*

<u>Ingredients</u>

- ✓ 1 tablespoon of pumpkin seeds
- ✓ ½ cup of frozen pineapples
- ✓ ½ cup of frozen bananas
- ✓ 1 cup of unsweetened yoghurt.

<u>Directions</u>

- ✓ Pour your frozen pineapples inside a blender
- ✓ Put your bananas and pumpkin seeds
- ✓ Supply your yoghurt

- ✓ And blend everything together until smooth
- ✓ Pour in a glass and serve with ice.

Carrots Smoothie

This orange beauty will not just leave your skin layer glowing, as well as your immunity high, but it additionally does wonders for sexual health.

Studies show that men who eat carrots at least 4 times weekly show a rise in sperm fertility and sexual prowess inside the bedroom.

Ingredients

- ✓ 1 cup of diced carrots
- ✓ 1 medium apple
- ✓ ½ cup of diced pineapples
- ✓ 10 grams of ginger

Direction

- ✓ Pour your diced or shredded carrots into the blender
- ✓ Put your diced apples and pineapples

- ✓ Put in a glass of water as well as your grated gingers
- ✓ Blend your ingredients together until smooth
- ✓ Pour in a glass and then add cubes of ice which are prepared to drink.

Banana Booster

Two things one thinks of when it comes to bananas: smiles and undoubtedly penises. Bananas are aphrodisiac, providing long-term energy and stamina as well as stimulating the production of serotonin, which helps improve sleep and elevate mood. Adding chia seeds into the mix transforms this smoothie into an energy tonic that moistens yin energy *(feminine)*. Beyond these benefits, this dairy-free smoothie is jam-packed with the *feel-good chemical* **dopamine**, along with *zinc, magnesium and vitamin B6*, all shown to have effects on improving mood.

Blend the first three ingredients until smooth, bring the rest of the ingredients, blend and serve. This recipe serves one.

- ✓ ¼ cup raw cashews
- ✓ 2 pitted dates
- ✓ 1¼ c water
- ✓ 1 frozen banana
- ✓ 1 Tbsp chia seeds
- ✓ Handful of ice

Chocolate Peanut Butter Smoothie

Cocoa beans have always been used to improve libido. This aphrodisiac was so potent that it had been actually prescribed by physicians in the 1800s as a reliable remedy for a minimal libido. Chocolate was known as *"food for the gods"* by the **Aztecs** due to its capability to release dopamine, which is the brain's pleasure chemical. With the combination of *peanut butter and banana*, this smoothie is usually filled up with *vitamin D and B, zinc and contains the amino acid L-arginine* which promotes healthy blood flow to sex organs.

Combine these ingredients and blend until it becomes smooth for an energizing smoothie which is able to maintain you up in more ways than one!

- ✓ 1¼ c skim milk
- ✓ ¼ c plain Greek yogurt
- ✓ 1 Tbsp natural peanut butter
- ✓ 1 Tbsp cocoa powder
- ✓ 1 frozen banana
- ✓ Handful of ice

Strawberry Stress Buster

Red may be the color of passion, so when it involves the red hue of strawberries, these ovary-shaped aphrodisiac fruits are thought to increase passion and promote healthy blood circulation to the mind and extremities. The bitterness in these berries also indicates their capability to activate the liver in removing hormones that the body no longer needs. By combining strawberries with magnesium-rich almond milk, the agitation and sleeplessness are combated while providing an ample dose of vitamin C. Adding vanilla into the mix brings awareness to the genitals, as this potent herb is known to cause *urethral irritation*.

Combine the next measurements of ingredients and blend until it is smooth for any flavorful and beneficial afternoon pick-me-up.

- ✓ 1½ c unsweetened almond milk
- ✓ 1 c frozen strawberries
- ✓ 1 tsp vanilla extract

Chocolate Strawberry Banana Smoothie

Ingredients

- ✓ 1/2 frozen banana
- ✓ 1/4 cup strawberries, fresh or frozen
- ✓ 1/4 cup peaches, fresh or frozen
- ✓ 1 tablespoon raw pumpkin seeds
- ✓ 1 tablespoon chocolates (70-percent cocoa or even more)
- ✓ 1/2 cup chocolates almond milk
- ✓ 1/2 cup cool water
- ✓ 1/8 teaspoon ginger

Directions

Pour ingredients into a blender, blend until smooth, and revel in!

Chapter 3
Foods that enhances Sexual drive
Chili Peppers

Chili Peppers-healthy and delicious aphrodisiacs

Maintain things hot and spicy with this aphrodisiac. *Chili peppers* support the chemical capsaicin, which helps increase circulation, heart rate, induce sweating, and raise the sensitivity of nerve endings. Capsaicin can be an all-natural irritant, so it's recognized to result in a stinging, tingling sensation - adding a spark and sizzle to every kiss.

Avocado

Avocado-healthy and delicious aphrodisiacs

This rich and creamy fruit continues to be considered an aphrodisiac dating back to the Aztec time. Back then it had been because of its sensuous pear shape, and even though that shape still helps avocado look appealing, its high degrees of vitamin E is actually what it's known for. Vitamin E is thought to support one, and maintain youthful vigor and energy, as well as assist in lubrication.

Raw Chocolate

The entire world loves chocolate. There have been 3.97 million a lot of cocoa beans stated in 2008-2009. That's incredible there should be something to it that it's almost everyone's favorite treat, but magic is in the beans (that aren't sweet) not the sugar. Chocolate originates from cocoa beans. Raw cocoa was also termed the nourishment in the gods by the Aztecs. It's a superfood with tons of antioxidants and stimulating chemicals such as phenylethylamine which stimulates the sense of excitement and well-being. The Journal of Sexual Medicine published a study that found that women who enjoy a piece of chocolate on a daily basis have a more active sex life than those you don't.

Dark Chocolate

Dark Chocolate healthy and delicious aphrodisiacs
Another reason chocolate makes an ideal gift to your Valentine! Chocolate contains *L-arginine*, an amino acid that increases nitric oxide and promotes blood circulation to sexual organs for men and women. L-arginine may also assist in sensation and satisfaction. Additionally,

chocolate also includes phenylethylamine and theobromine. The compound theobromine might help you feel activated and excited, and phenylethylamine helps improves moods by increasing serotonin levels.

Bananas

Bananas-healthy and delicious aphrodisiacs

Bananas are not just nice and delicious, they are also packed with vitamin B and potassium, which are two essential elements in the production of sex hormones. Bananas are also filled with chelating nutrients, which help your body absorb essential nutrients and so are therefore thought to raise the male libido.

Honey

Honey is a healthy and delicious aphrodisiacs

Honey does a lot more than sweeten; it's also an excellent way to obtain boron, which includes been shown to greatly help stimulate estrogen production in women and testosterone production in men. Honey can be thought to increase nitric oxide levels, which may be the chemical released during arousal. No wonder it's a term of endearment!

Watermelon

Watermelon-healthy and delicious aphrodisiacs

This hydrating fruit contains citrulline, a plant nutrient recognized to benefit the cardiovascular and disease-fighting capability. ***Citrulline*** can be thought to work similarly to Viagra, for the reason that it relaxes arteries and improves blood circulation.

Pine Nuts

Pine nuts do a lot more than put in a zest to some dish, they are able to also reportedly assist with sexual stamina in men. That is because of the high zinc content, which protects against impotence and infertility.

Arugula

arugula-healthy and delicious aphrodisiacs

Arugula offers reportedly have been used as an aphrodisiac because of the initial century. Research shows that this trace minerals and antioxidants in dark, leafy greens are crucial for sexual health because they help block environmental contaminants that may negatively affect our libidos.

Figs

Figs-Healthy and delicious aphrodisiacs

Figs have already been around for years and were Cleopatra's favorite fruit. The ancient Greeks associated them with love and fertility, and with justification! Figs are saturated in flavonoids and antioxidants, that may assist in sexual stamina.

Strawberries

Strawberries-Healthy and Delicious Aphrodisiacs

Strawberries dipped in chocolate will be the ultimate Valentine's Day treat! Maybe it is because strawberries are abundant with folic acid and vitamin C, which may help increase sperm fertility and improve sperm motility.

Pomegranates

Pomegranate-Aphrodisiacs.

The abundance of antioxidants in pomegranates give this fruit its aphrodisiac qualities. Antioxidants protect the liner of arteries, allowing more blood to course through them, which helps increase genital sensitivity.

Maca

Maca is really a trendy superfood from Peru. And it deserves to shine: It grows 4,100 m above sea level in the Andes. Maca may be the energizing and revitalizing superfood of the Incas, who revered it because of its aphrodisiac qualities and wide-ranging advantages to the hormonal system. It's been used for 2000 years and which can make you a genuine Incan warrior during intercourse, therefore the legend tells. Personally, when I have a spoonful of Maca, I get horny just about immediately! And at the top, it has plenty of healing potential too.

Cinnamon

Hormone imbalance is normally the root cause with regards to a minimal mojo. Cinnamon is among the popular spices for Christmas but also used since ancient occasions to improve sexual interest.

Yes, you should use one that you currently have within your kitchen or will get to buy nearby. Ideally organic.

Ashwagandha

This one is fantastic too. Started in India, utilized for a large number of years by Ayurvedic practitioners. It's also known as the Indian Ginseng. One study demonstrates *Ashwagandha* stimulates an enzyme referred to as nitric oxide, this can help with the dilating of arteries to the genital organs. It's a brilliant high antioxidant that may increase your libido but also your disease fighting capability.

Coconut Oil

Without a doubt, this oil is hyped days past, they have incredible sexy use cases, from lubrication to breast massage oil to beautiful skin. Some coconut fanatics say that it could improve your libido, which might be because of antioxidants in the oil that assist combat free radicals that may result in a lowered libido.

Almonds

Selenium might help with infertility issues and, with vitamin E, can help heart health. Zinc is actually a mineral that helps produce men's sex hormones and may boost libido. Blood circulation is very important to your sex organs, so choosing good fats, like the omega-3 fatty acids within almonds, is a genuinely good idea.

Chapter 4
How to Improve Your Sex Life

So before you pop those sex enhancement pill, remember nature includes a healthier alternative, that is included with no risk to the heart. Turns out, plenty of women, plus some men too, suffer from sexual dysfunction or simply deficiencies in interest in sex. Increasingly more, some women don't even have a sexual prime. They're perennially exhausted, and with reserves running low, sex may be the very first thing to go.

Moms of small children have become often less thinking about sex than their partners. Husbands are frustrated and wonder what happened to the energetic woman they married. (Have just a little patience, men. It could perfectly be temporary. Sort of an extended temporary, I understand, but nonetheless, it's a season.) Another growing phenomenon is low testosterone in men. A lot of men possess less need for sex now than they did 50 years back. Research shows that high blood pressure, raised cholesterol, diabetes, and obesity lower testosterone, and (surprise!) many of these conditions are increasing.

Depression and anxiety will also be increasing, even though these circumstances are libido-killers in themselves, the medications used to take care of them have the normal side-effect of causing sexual dysfunction. The urinary tract, which modulates your hormones (and for that reason, your libido), is easily disrupted. Besides medications, endocrine disruptors in the surroundings, home products, as well as our food supply are recognized to cause a wide variety of reproductive problems, including low libido.

Nutritional Tips for Boosting Libido

We have several tips for all those experiencing low libido, or possibly it's your lover whose libido doesn't match yours. I'm likely to focus on the DON'Ts and get to the DOs:

Ditch Endocrine-Disrupting Plastics

Don't drink out of plastic containers or microwave stuff in plastic (or, heaven forbid, styrofoam).

Don't Drink Plain Tap Water - Avoid Fluoride and Chlorine

Get yourself a carbon filter overall water system in your house. Get yourself a reverse osmosis filtering, at the very least. On top of that would be to own R.O. water and a water ionizer.

Don't Eat Soy!

Soy and soy-based products have the potential to wreak havoc on your own libido. Most soy inside the U.S. are certainly genetically altered, but worse, processed soy products mimic estrogen in the torso and disrupt the standard hormone function. Don't use soy milk or any other processed soy products; occasionally, smaller amounts of organic miso, edamame, tofu, Nama shoyu, or Bragg's are okay.

Read your labels! You will find soy protein isolate and soy lecithin and twelve other prepared soy fractions in everything boxed, everything canned, and everything manufactured by humans nowadays, including virtually all bread products. Everything accumulates, so cut it out of your daily diet.

Quit Using Chemical-based Skin Products

Make sure the products you utilize on your skin are completely natural to improve your libido. Putting it on your own skin is equivalent to eating it. Your skin layer is a full-time income, breathing organ, and it requires what you placed on it into the bloodstream. Make a shift to the items you placed on your skin layer is only natural. My moisturizer is organic coconut oil.

The types of Foods to eat for an Improved Sex Life

Eat Whole-Food Plants

Consuming whole food plants offers you more energy that may lead to improved sex life. A quart of a green smoothie is among the easiest methods for getting 7-10 portions of fruits & vegetables every day.

Among my biggest surprises on paper, the Green Smoothies Diet was discovering that lots of people that drink green smoothies regularly, within my report of 175 people, experience higher libido. (The sex-drive statistic, if you ask me at least, pertains to both vigor and interest in an exceedingly intense, personal reference to other people. In ways, it's just producing your hormones balanced and healthier, and that's an excellent stage too, I believe a higher libido is an all-natural state.) And when plants are everything you eat the majority of, weight loss almost inevitable.

Actually being 10 pounds over your normal weight can vary noticeably affect libido or trigger low libido. It may seem depressing libido is basically because you don't look sexy or uninhibited when you've got love handles or thigh flab. That's only part of it.

A significant part is a fact that feeling sexy and energetic does result in you being your very self-in in all ways. On the other hand, need to turn the lights off, avoid certain areas of the body being visible, or fretting about insecurities, results in nothing good in the bedroom. The other part is how simply a supplementary 10lbs. truly depresses circulation and endocrine functions. You truly need those functions once and for all lovin'.

Whenever your energy is depleted, since it always is going to be on the typical American Diet diet, you lose the sexual interest and stamina you once had. Sexual dysfunction happens in the same manner all degenerative diseases do: it is linked to lifestyle choices. Your reproductive system, in the end, is suffering from similar things your cardiac, circulatory, and endocrine systems are. All of them are inextricably linked because they are all part of 1 complex organs.

Add these to Your Green;

It's half for you personally and a half for your lover. Here they may be:

Maca

Maca may be the "Peruvian ginseng," a root vegetable prized from the Incans for a large number of years because of its capability to improve athletic endurance and sexual stamina.

Bee pollen

Look what it can for the queen bee! Bee pollen is normally a robust aphrodisiac. Make an effort one grain to be sure you're not allergic and two grains the very next day. Put a spoonful from it within your libido-boosting smoothie when you've ascertained you don't have a sensitivity to it. In addition, it includes a potentially helpful influence on seasonal allergies and immune function! Bee pollen can provide a naturally powerful boost for your libido.

Celery

Yes, the vegetable I affectionately prefer to say originates from the cardboard family. Put it inside your sex smoothie recipe where you won't see it because it contains androsterone, a precursor to pheromones that positively affect the sexual behavior of your lover.

Eat Foods Containing Zinc

Zinc blocks the enzyme that converts testosterone (in charge of libido) into estrogen. Make an effort to also get kidney and lima beans, spinach, some flax, garlic, and peanuts.

Review the Drugs You Take

Many over-the-counter and prescription medications suppress libido or causes additional sexual dysfunction.

Common culprits are the following:
- ✓ Antihistamines
- ✓ Antidepressants
- ✓ Contraceptive pills or patches
- ✓ Hair thinning treatments
- ✓ Beta-blockers
- ✓ Opioids
- ✓ Medical marijuana

Try turning to a thing that doesn't experience effects on your own libido. Even better, address the primary cause of the problem and that means you can eventually ditch the meds.

Embrace Change of Time

Some people are simply just interested in sex each day, instead of during the night. It's a truism that lots of individuals are either "nighttime people" or "morning people." There's nothing wrong with that. You merely may need to compromise if your lover may be the opposite.

Consult Bioidentical Hormone Specialist

Women obtaining a full blood-panel workup to learn if progesterone or female testosterone may be the base of the problem. Just a little progesterone or hormone cream may work wonders. (However, you want this only when it's warranted from your test outcomes!) Testosterone cream is suitable only when you are 40 or older.

Please get these only from a bioidentical practitioner. The substances aren't identical to what the body makes. They can be harmful and could involve some symptom-abatement results for a while, but they may also be connected with negative unwanted effects and disease risk. Additional remedies your natural care practitioner may recommend, like DHEA or flax oil, could possibly be very easily located at a health grocery.

Much better than Pills

Each day we are been bombarded with ads recommending male and female medications and herbal treatments for sexual dysfunction. They are actually used in an instant, short-term fix, however, they do not get to solve the main problem, plus they come at a price. Not merely are they expensive, however, they create a growing set of serious unwanted effects such as gastrointestinal problems, memory and vision loss and hearing impairment. Additionally, they hinder the additional medications we take.

So your investment pills! Start juicing for a wholesome and natural enhancement of the sexual experience! Here is a review of the foodstuffs that contain the best concentration of sexually stimulating nutrients - all proven by nutritional research!

Chapter 5

Foods to stay away from

These food types lower libido in men and women, and really should be avoided to be able to ensure the healthy maintenance of your sex life:

Sugar

Processed sugar isn't only unhealthy, it diminishes testosterone in men, thus lowering male libido.

Trans-Fats

Not merely are trans fats nutritionally unhealthy, they lower blood flow and therefore diminish sexual ability in men and women.

Canned Foods

Most cans are lined with *'BPA,'* a substance which, in high levels of exposure have been reported to cause erection dysfunction just as much as four times more regularly in men who consume canned foods frequently. Search for this ***"BPA FREE"*** label on cans.

Soy

Soy lowers libido in men by diminishing testosterone because of the occurrence of estrogen-like compounds.

Salt

Huge amounts of sodium are a source of impotence problems that even medication can not undo.

Alcohol

Though it diminishes inhibition and lessens stress, alcohol lowers our capability to perform and also to get sexually satisfied. Fresh juiced fruits & vegetables with added nuts and spices aren't just a smart way to increase your well-being, strengthen muscle, and reduce weight. Sure combinations, as in the above list, will truly improve your sex life. No matter what your actual age, juicing is among the best methods to have significantly more fun.

Chapter 6

Understanding Women Erogenous Zones

A woman's sexual organs are called the **genitalia**, meaning the genital organs. They contain the **vagina** as well as the **vulva**. The vagina can be an internal tube-shaped cavity connecting the exterior towards the cervix from the uterus. The cervix may be the opening for the uterus. The vagina is separate from your vulva. The vulva is usually beyond your body and includes all of the outer genitals you can view whenever you open your legs and appear before the mirror. The looks in the vulva may differ quite a bit between different women, and each one of these variations is believed reasonable.

It could be compared to additional anatomical variations, such as some women have big hips, some have small hips, some possess a big nose, some have a little nose, some have large pendulous breasts, some have perky compact breasts plus some experience hardly any breast tissue.

The Vulva

The term vulva means covering, which is suitable since it covers and protects the opening of the vagina plus the opening towards the bladder. The opening for the bladder's exit tube is named the ***urethral meatus,*** which is where urine exits. The vulva includes the following parts:

- ***The outer lips (the labia majora):*** Your skin of the external mouth contains hair roots and glands that secrete sweat and a waxy liquid called *sebum*.
- ***The inner lips (the labia minora):*** They are smaller and thinner compared to the exterior lip area, and so are hairless. The looks and size of the inner lips may differ significantly between women.
- The edges of both lips contain tiny glands that secrete oily fluid necessary to the fitness of the vagina opening. These glands can appear as very small white lumps, that is normal.
- ***The vestibule:*** this is the region that exists between inner lip area. At the center of the vestibule, we find the openings of the vagina and urinary system. The vestibule comes with extremely rich blood and nerve supply and, during sexual arousal, the

vestibule and inner lips become engorged with blood.

- The ***clitoris*** is normally viewed by women like a little raised firm nub of tissue near the top of the inner lips. It looks small, right? Yes, it can, and you'll think you have already been short-changed in comparison to men, however, in fact, the clitoris is a lot bigger than the 1/4 inch tip you can view and experience. This nub of tissue is named the *glans clitoris*.

The glans clitoris is mounted on a shaft around 1 inch long that connects to your pubic bone, which shaft divides into 2 roots referred to as *crura* that put on the pelvic bones. You can not possibly see the shaft along with the roots because they are included in tissue. The clitoris comes by a large number of nerve endings, which will make it extremely sensitive to touch. Some women discover that direct stimulation from the glans clitoris is too intense and almost painful, plus they realize that it feels far better if their partner gently stimulates the shaft in the clitoris. In case your clitoris is incredibly sensitive, ask your lover to be very gentle as he touches you lightly, especially in the first instance.

Many women can reach orgasm from the stimulation of the clitoris either by their partner or by their fingers or perhaps a vibrator. That is a very important thing, as over fifty percent of most women hardly achieve orgasm from vaginal intercourse.

Do you know why? Men have no idea of this, and perhaps it is hard to allow them to consider it.

During sexual arousal, the clitoris swells to around double its size since it offers such an enormous blood circulation. Thus a wholesome blood flow is vital to an excellent sexual response. Blood can flow into and from the clitoris, causing it to change in size, which enables some women to get multiple orgasms. Things that decrease the blood supply, such as diabetes, high blood pressure, or smoking can lessen a woman's ability to experience clitoral orgasms. Testosterone therapy can raise the size and sensitivity of the clitoris, and women with surprisingly low testosterone levels may have problems reaching orgasm.

The G Spot

The **G-spot** is famous but also controversial, as there continues to be a whole lot of discussion concerning where it really is and when it indeed occurs. Couples have already told me that it is lots of fun looking for the G spot! This famous spot is regarded as probably the most sexually sensitive as well as the most arousing spot for a few women, however, not for all women.

So, where can the G spot be located?

It is regarded as a location of tissue in the low front wall from the vagina just close to the urethra. This region is smooth rather than wrinkly, just like the vagina. Some researchers believe that the G spot may be underneath the area of the clitoris when it's activated or pressured through the leading wall of the vagina.

The G spot may be partly within the tissue just within the skin with the *vestibule* - that is called the bulb on the *vestibule*. This tissue comes with extremely rich blood circulation, so when blood flows into this tissue, the vestibule enlarges and stiffens, you can say just like a type of female erection.

The G spot is evident if a woman is sexually aroused, so don't embark on a finding expedition if you're not searching for the G spot by rubbing along the low front wall within the vagina with two fingers, a dildo or vibrator. Remember, it isn't high up in the vagina close to the cervix. Some women report experiencing incredible sensations through the G spot if indeed they hold rear entry vaginal sex or if they're together with their partner. Some women haven't found their G spot but enjoy a wonderful sex life with many orgasms, so do not worry if you fail to think it is - we all are different, and that's normal.

Orgasms

You might be surprised, and perhaps relieved, to learn that over fifty percent of most women usually do not reach orgasm with vaginal intercourse. This means that if sex is fixed to just the insertion of the penis into the vagina and thrusting of the penis in the vagina, most women won't experience an orgasm quite simply they'll not climax.

Was God a male chauvinist?

I don't believe so; it's that there are various ways to come with orgasm, and women will vary in the manner they achieve the elusive orgasm. It's just normal to vary.

The standard differences are:

- Some women have a lot more difficulty achieving orgasms than others, and we don't always know why.
- Women achieve orgasm through different mechanisms.
- Some women have multiple orgasms routinely, while others do not have several throughout a sexual encounter.
- The intensity of orgasms may differ a lot in a single woman at differing times and between different women.

It might be just a little whimper, or it might be an intensely enjoyable volcano. Though it feels good with an orgasm, especially a rigorous one which releases tension, it isn't essential to provide an orgasm every time you have sexual intercourse; indeed, it isn't a norm for some women. You will be sexually satisfied even though you don't have an orgasm. You will find no rules to check out, no template you should attempt to emulate.

What physical adjustments happen within you during an orgasm?

The founders of present-day sexual medicine, Masters, and Johnson, first described the four stages of sexual response in ladies in 1966. These stages gave us an overall physiological picture; however, understand that every woman differs, if you do not match these stages exactly, don't worry, you are healthy. The main thing about sex can be to take pleasure from it; it's designed for fun and relaxation. If you try too much to be always a femme fatale or even to possess multiple orgasms, you may pass up out, as you'll have a lot in your mind rather than enough within your pelvis.

The First Stage - Excitement

During stage one, you feel aroused which causes the vulva to swell with blood - that is called *engorgement*.

An all-natural chemical called **Nitric Oxide (NO)** is stated in the walls of the blood vessels providing the vulva an increased amounts. **NO** is a powerful dilator of arteries, so when the arteries grow wider, the blood circulation increases dramatically, plus the vulva swells. This whole area feels full, warm, plus much more reactive. The fluid then starts to be secreted from the liner with the vagina and vulva to create the essential lubrication. The quantity of fluid secreted may differ a whole lot, and that's the reason lubricants are occasionally required.

The top area of the vagina expands from its normally collapsed state to some cavity wide enough to support an erect penis. The uterus and cervix rise inside the pelvic cavity to create room for the erect penis. Your body produces extra adrenalin, which in turn causes the pulse rate to improve, the blood circulation pressure to go up; the muscles become poised and mental excitement is heightened. This is the best time for your lover to excite your clitoris because you are prepared to respond.

You may want to teach your lover to wait until you are in this mood before your clitoris is touched, as though it's done prematurely or too roughly, you won't feel right and even could be unpleasant. *We have to teach men about foreplay; for most men, it isn't instinctual;* they have got to either find out about it inside a magazine or talked with their mates or experimented on other women who were non-communicative. Your partner is going to be relieved to get informative tips from you.

You might have noticed the joke.

A female asks a guy, "Just how long does it take for a female to orgasm?"

The person replies, *"Who cares!"*

Thankfully most men aren't like this; however, there are a few cultures where only men's desires and satisfaction are believed necessary.

A lot of women test out a vibrator during their life and advantages include

- Studying your own body and its responses,
- The capability to have the ability to do something positive about your arousal when you wish to,
- Spare batteries are cheap and uncomplicated,
- They have got an on/off switch you can control,

- They don't fall asleep by the end of stage one.

The Second Stage - Plateau

When the initial stage is complete along with the vulva is engorged with blood, the excitement starts to level off. The tissues around the low vagina swell, thus narrowing the vagina and squeeze the penis, which feels good to both partners. Through the plateau phase, the uterus is pushed up further as well as the upper area of the vagina expands way more that the penis can thrust in more in-depth. The labia minora (inner lips) expand and swell changing color into a deeper red. The plateau phase varies in duration, and a female may return into the excitement phase for some time and then back to the plateau phase.

The Third Stage - Orgasm

When orgasm occurs, there is certainly intense pleasure associated with contractions on the muscles around the vagina and in the tissues between your vagina and anus. For most women, orgasm can't be made by vaginal

If you have regular sex with your partner, the recurrent release of oxytocin keeps you bonded and attached to your partner. Oxytocin helps couples stay together, physically, and emotionally.

Support For Orgasms

Irrespective of where you fall in the standard spectral range of sexual response, you may increase your orgasms. Indeed with the proper technique from your partner or yourself via masturbation, you might be in a position to achieve some multiple orgasms.

Almost all women masturbate; they'll use either their fingers or even a vibrator. This is quite healthy and normal, and it is not a sign of any character weakness or sexual depravity.

Masturbation will never lead to an increase in diseases of the vulva and pelvic organs. Regular orgasms achieved through masturbation may be healthy and promote better circulation of blood to the pelvic organs and strengthen the pelvic floor muscles.

Many normal women begin to masturbate during their teen years, and this way, they get to know themselves and can avoid having sexual intercourse before they are ready and before they have adequate contraception. Some women do not begin to explore the feeling of masturbation and clitoral stimulation until much later in life, say in their late 20s or 30s. In these women, it is often an incompetent or selfish lover that leaves them frustrated and wondering, *"Is this all there is?"* that prompts them to masturbate. The orgasm they give themselves will relieve their sexual frustration. Many women will need help to orgasm, especially as they get older, if they have hormonal imbalances or if they have health problems. The sex hormones *estrogen, progesterone, and testosterone* prepare and prime your genital organs for sex. They make you interested and ready to receive.

Low levels of estrogen cause the vulva and vagina to be thin and shrink (atrophy), and their membranes dry out. *This makes you too fragile for sex. Adequate levels of all three sex hormones keep your vagina and vulva robust, plumper, supple, and moist - they make you responsive and inviting.* They also increase blood flow to the vulva and increase sensitivity. *Testosterone* makes you the warrior woman and gives you the confidence and desire to conquer the man in your life, at least in bed. However, it can also promote emotional strength as well. *Hormonal creams and oxytocin* can make a huge difference and can turn the vast majority of women of all ages into orgasmic creatures.

You need to be an excellent communicator with your sex partner and, if you feel frustrated, tell your partner the exact technique you need them to use for you to achieve satisfaction. If poor communication is a persistent problem, consult a professional sex therapist together.

Sexual Desire

The desire to have sex is categorized as **libido,** which varies enormously between women. Some women have a continual need for sex and are always ready for their partners. Other women do not think about sex very much and are more focused on their career, children, or family. Sexual desire generally reduces with age, although older women often find that hormone replacement therapy can rekindle their interest.

It is quite normal for libido to be higher at the beginning of a new relationship. Once you get to know each other and have conquered your mate, so to speak, the intensity of sexual desire may gradually wane.

Your environment has a significant effect on your libido, and women often find that their libido resurfaces like the Phoenix when they go away with their partner on holiday away from family and work. Yes, you need more holidays together! Some women have a naturally low libido, and this does not worry them; in other words, low libido is not an issue or a medical problem unless it worries you.

Sexual desire in women is often affected by the physical and mental status of their partner. If your partner smells like a brewery, or an ashtray, is drug-affected, has body odour, or is grumpy, well, then reading a magazine or eating an apple pie with ice cream has got to be sexier than sex!

Let's face it; women want to feel special if our partner wants to have sex with us we are worth their effort!

Chapter 7

Sources of Poor Libido in Women

After menopause, nearly all women lose adequate production of *estrogen and progesterone,* which may reduce sexual desire and the ability to enjoy sex. The loss of estrogen causes the tissues of the vagina and vulva to shrink and dry out, and the clitoris becomes smaller and less sensitive. Indeed, the clitoris may become tender to touch so that foreplay becomes uncomfortable.

The loss of estrogen causes a loss of vaginal secretions. The loss of progesterone causes reduced sexual desire and may also cause mood changes. After menopause, the amount of testosterone produced by the ovaries and fat tissues varies a lot and this is why blood tests to measure the level of testosterone are so important to choose the types and amounts of hormones required in the cream. Some women produce plenty of testosterone after menopause and thus do not need any testosterone in their prescriptions. Other women may need testosterone in their prescriptions if their blood tests show low levels. Testosterone is a very important hormone for libido and sexual response, and, in women with low levels, it is essential to prescribe some natural testosterone, either in the form of a cream or lozenge. Testosterone can make women more sexually assertive and sexually confident, and indeed too much testosterone can result in excessive sexual drive in some women.

Menopause

The human female may be the only creature recognized to live a lot longer than her sex glands and reproductive capacity; with this context, we have become dissimilar to men, so no wonder older women need just a little support to rev up in the bedroom. When their ovaries run out of eggs (follicles), the production of progesterone ceases entirely, and estrogen levels become very low.

The average age of menopause is 50 years, but a significant percentage of women go through early menopause, and their eggs are totally gone before they get to 40 years, this is called premature menopause. I have had patients who go through menopause in their 20s, and these women need a lot more help with hormone replacement. Before the menopause, the majority of estrogen is produced by ovaries. After the menopause, when the ovaries are devoid of useful eggs, the vast majority of estrogen is produced away from ovaries in fat tissue. I have found that thinner women often have more pronounced estrogen deficiency symptoms.

The blood test for menopause is a measurement of the ***Follicle Stimulating Hormone (FSH),*** and if this is elevated, you are menopausal, and you have no fertile eggs. If your *FSH levels are over **30 IU/L*** on two separate blood tests, you are deemed menopausal, and the higher your FSH levels, the lower your estrogen and progesterone levels will be. The FSH is produced by the pituitary gland and acts to stimulate the ovaries back into the production of the sex hormones *estrogen and progesterone.*

In post-menopausal women it is not uncommon to see very high levels of FSH around 100 to 200 IU/L, which are coming from the pituitary gland, and this means your estrogen levels will be very low. These high levels of FSH will not be successful in stimulating your ovaries back to work because they no longer have any eggs left in them to respond to the FSH. Your ovaries have closed shop or gone on strike forever, and thus; these high levels of FSH achieve nothing but do serve as an accurate blood test for menopause.

All women wish to know if they are truly menopausal and have to know their FSH level to find out this. In case your FSH level is extremely high, you have no fertile eggs and will no longer have to worry about contraception; this may improve your libido! If you are taking the oral contraceptive pill, you will need to stop taking it for several months before having a blood test for menopause; otherwise, the test will be inaccurate. So don't waste your money having blood tests for your hormone levels while you are still taking the oral contraceptive pill. Many doctors do not realize this, so it's wise to inform yourself.

Progesterone deficiency

Progesterone is a sex hormone that's made by the feminine ovaries through the latter half of the menstrual period and in huge quantities by the placenta during pregnancy. A lot of women begin to become progesterone deficient within their late 30s and 40s, way before they reach menopause. By the time these women reach menopause, their levels may only be 20% of the youthful progesterone amounts. Progesterone provides anti-aging properties and is also important for libido. Progesterone exerts a relaxing effect and may promote emotional contentment and stableness.

The brain offers receptors for progesterone, which is definitely why natural hormones can be so beneficial for emotional disorders. If you find your mood and sex drive lower during the one to two weeks before your menstrual bleeding commences, then you will probably benefit from natural progesterone. Progesterone deficiency is very common in women today because they often delay pregnancy to later in life and have fewer pregnancies. Progesterone deficiency can cause unpleasant moods such as *anxiety, irritability, irrational thinking, reduced libido, and depression*. Progesterone deficiency can also cause physical health problems such as heavy and/or painful menstrual bleeding, endometriosis, fibroids, increased risk of cancer, premenstrual headaches, polycystic ovarian syndrome, and unexplained infertility.

The use of natural progesterone was first advocated back in the 1960s by *Dr. Katharina Dalton*, an English physician who was somewhat of a **'PMS Guru'**. Natural progesterone can be beneficial in reducing the following problems;

- Depression, anxiety, and mood changes
- Iron deficiency and fatigue
- Heavy menstrual bleeding
- Menstrual pain
- Pelvic congestion, pain and bloating
- Breast pain
- Poor libido
- Insomnia

It is important to realize that Dr. Dalton recommended the use of natural progesterone, which has a chemical structure identical to the progesterone produced by the ovaries. Natural progesterone is made in the laboratory from the plant hormone called ***diosgenin*** found in *soybeans and sweet potatoes (yams),* b*ecause natural* progesterone is identical to the progesterone produced by the ovaries, it is called a ***bio-identical hormone***.

Unfortunately, doctors often prescribe strong synthetic brands of progesterone called *'progestogens,'* mistakenly believing that they can own the same effect as natural progesterone. This is simply not true, and synthetic progesterone will usually make most of the symptoms of PMS much worse.

Many of these synthetic progestogens are derived from male (testosterone-like) synthetic hormones and so may cause side effects such as increased appetite, depression, irritability, weight gain, fluid retention, acne, greasy skin, and increased cholesterol. These synthetic progestogen hormones attach to the natural progesterone receptors found throughout the body and brain, but they cannot switch on all these receptors. Only natural progesterone can turn on all the progesterone receptors just as a key turns and releases a lock. So you can understand that synthetic progestogens will not have the same beneficial effect as natural progesterone, and indeed, many women feel more depressed and tired when they take them.

However, synthetic progestogens are effective at reducing heavy menstrual bleeding and some types of gynaecological problems such as endometriosis. Progesterone deficiency is common in:
- Young women with menstrual problems,
- Women after childbirth where it is associated with postnatal depression,
- Women with cyclical mood disorders and bipolar illness,
- Women with thyroid problems such as Hashimoto's thyroiditis or Grave's disease,
- Women after a miscarriage,
- Peri-menopausal women.

How do I know if I am progesterone deficient?

It is not generally necessary or useful to do blood or salivary tests to prove that a deficiency of progesterone exists. This is because a doctor who understands progesterone can tell from the history of the patient if they are deficient. Keeping a menstrual calendar of symptoms to show your doctor can help to pinpoint the premenstrual exacerbation. Symptoms of progesterone deficiency include:

- Heavy and/or painful periods
- Poor libido
- Insomnia
- Premenstrual headaches
- Fibroids, endometriosis or adenomyosis in the uterus
- Unexplained infertility
- Polycystic ovarian syndrome
- Premenstrual syndrome/moodiness and postnatal depression
- Iron insufficiency
- Infrequent or irregular periods
- Hair loss
- Breast pain and/or lumpiness

The good news is that natural progesterone therapy can often alleviate these symptoms in women of all ages. Thus one would think that natural progesterone is commonly prescribed for these diverse and common problems. In reality, however, few doctors prescribe natural progesterone because it cannot be patented by drug companies. Thus drug companies do not promote it or educate doctors about its make, uses or benefits. This is a pity and results in much-unneeded suffering for women. In my opinion, the best way to administer natural progesterone is in the form of a cream that is rubbed onto the skin.

Polycystic ovarian syndrome

Hormonal imbalances can drive women to accomplish a variety of extreme things, especially premenstrually and through the postnatal period, and these exact things could be most out of proportion.

Fatigue

Lack of vigor is usually a common reason behind disinterest in sex because making love does take time and attempt, particularly if you are to accomplish it well and revel in it. In the event that you are too tired, it is possible to understand that you'll rather utilize the time to rest or sleep. Common reasons for fatigue in women are iron deficiency, depression, sleep disorders, and the excessive busyness of being a mother, domestic goddess, and breadwinner. Poor diet, lack of exercise, and general poor health produce fatigue, which can drain away your sexual energy.

Many women tell me that if they go away on holiday just with their husband, their libido returns, and they enjoy fulfilling sex. Life is just too busy and complicated these days for many women to have the luxury of time and peace to be conscious of their sexuality.

Stress

I see a lot of women that have to spend the majority of their life looking after others. They could have elderly or sick parents, children with disabilities or behavioral problems, or possibly a husband, along with his own mental and emotional issues. Women tend to be the problem-solvers and rescuers, and in doing this, they often lose themselves. These angels often deserve a medal of honor, and I take my hat off to them every day. Hopefully, we can all be more aware of the sacrifices they make and enable them to have more respite.

Depression

The symptoms of depression often manifest as fatigue, lack of pleasure, and lack of desire for life and could insidiously develop over many years. Obviously, this may impair your psychological relationship together with your partner. Depression is certainly more common through the first year after childbirth when it's called postnatal depression, and around the time of menopause. Depression is often connected with feelings of low self-confidence and poor self-image and a lack of interest on the contrary sex.

Depression may be the consequence of a chemical imbalance in the brain with reduced levels of the brain's neuro-transmitters, namely ***dopamine, serotonin, and adrenalin***. Modern-day anti-depressants are effective at restoring the brain's levels of these neurotransmitters, and once they are back to normal, the symptoms of depression disappear. Anti-depressants may improve your emotional relationship with your partner, which may help your low libido; however, some anti-depressant medications make it impossible to achieve an orgasm. In this case, nasal oxytocin spray and natural hormone creams may help a lot.

The oral contraceptive pill

The oral contraceptive pill (OCP) will come in two forms. The most common form is named the combined oral contraceptive pill, and it possesses estrogen coupled with progesterone. The various form is recognized as the progesterone pill will not contain any estrogen. The combined oral contraceptive pill prevents over 99% of pregnancies, plus the progesterone pill is less effective like a contraceptive preventing around 95% of pregnancies. Both types of oral contraceptive pills contain synthetic hormones, as natural hormones aren't strong enough to avoid pregnancy.

The synthetic hormones within the contraceptive pill should be divided (metabolized) from the liver, whose procedure stimulates the liver to create greater levels of a protein called *Sex Hormone Binding Globulin (SHBG)*. **SHBG** functions to bind the naturally produced sex hormones in the torso, especially testosterone. Once a hormone is bound or mounted on SHBG it doesn't absolve to act in the torso which is thus inactivated. This decrease in the levels of free testosterone open to your body. It often reduces the libido because testosterone exerts a stimulating influence on the libido.

It isn't uncommon for women to complain of a lack of libido after they have already used the contraceptive pill for a number of months, which decreasing free testosterone may be the primary reason. The SHBG also binds the circulating degrees of estrogen, which can lead to vaginal dryness. The progesterone mini pill is normally less inclined to reduce the libido compared to the combined oral contraceptive pill. If you're using the contraceptive pill and discover its features reduced your libido or caused vaginal dryness, this is helped through the use of a cream combining natural estrogen and natural testosterone on the vulva. This cream must be used frequently.

Possible unwanted effects with the OCP consist of the following:

- Migraines, which may be severe
- Nausea and gallstones
- Water retention
- Putting on weight and bloating
- Reduced or total lack of libido
- Breast pain and lumpiness

- Blood clots and aggravation of varicose veins
- Elevation of blood circulation pressure
- Moodiness and depression in susceptible women.

When the OCP offers you side effects, you need to see your physician to try different brands of the OCP, because they contain various kinds of hormones. All of the hormones found in the OCP are synthetic, plus some women will struggle to tolerate the medial side effects. In women with heavy menstrual bleeding, an intrauterine contraceptive device called the **Mirena** could work effectively to lessen the menstrual bleeding to very light amounts.

The Mirena will not usually help overcome PMS symptoms such as mood disorders, and low libido, and in such instances, the natural progesterone cream could be used in combination with the *Mirena*. That is quite safe and will not hinder the contraceptive efficiency on the Mirena.

Note: It is imperative that ladies who want to prevent pregnancy and so are taking drugs or hormones to take care of low libido, sexual problems, or PMS have an adequate method of contraception.

Whenever a woman is taking the oral contraceptive pill, blood tests to gauge the natural degrees of sex hormones aren't beneficial or meaningful, as all they'll show is usually that you will be on the pill and that you have high degrees of SHBG and low degrees of estrogen and testosterone. In the event the OCP is destroying your libido, make an effort to get an alternative approach to contraception that won't lessen your sex hormones just as much, including the progestogen implant referred to as *Implanon* or the *Depot Provera injection*. Some women find a *MIRENA intrauterine contraceptive device* suits them well since it lightens the quantity of menstrual bleeding and will not reduce their very own natural hormone levels.

Medications that reduce libido

Many medications can hinder libido and sexual function but are unlikely to get the sole reason behind these problems. The condition that you are taking the medication can also be cutting down on your sexual function, and it could be difficult to learn what percentage from the problem is due to the medications set alongside the disease. In the event that you suspect a medication has reduced your libido, speak to your doctor as there are alternative medications you could take for the disease that won't affect your sex life.

The next medications can reduce libido:
- Drugs that affect the brain's degrees of *serotonin* and/or *dopamine*
- Drugs that increase Sex Hormone Binding *Globulin* (such as oral estrogens along with the oral contraceptive pill)
- Drugs that decrease the action of testosterone such as *cyproterone acetate*
- Some commonly prescribed antacids

The most frequent drugs recognized to reduce libido and orgasmic ability are anti-depressant medications. Antipsychotic medications utilized for treating schizophrenia or bipolar illness can reduce libido. Blood pressure medications (anti-hypertensives) may also reduce sexual function.

Vaginal odor and infection

The vaginal odor could be a switch off for both partners of the sexual relationship as much as bad breath could be; interestingly, by improving your gut health, you can improve both problems. Vaginal odor is frequently due to unfriendly bacteria such as *streptococci or Ecoli* growing in the vagina and these can originate on your skin around the anus and from your bowel. This problem is named **Bacterial Vaginosis (BV)**. Infection using the yeast organism called **candida** will not usually produce an odor but often causes a surplus vaginal discharge that's thick and white and could cause itchiness across the vulva.

Each one of these infections could be controlled by improving your disease fighting capability as well as your diet. Make an effort to eat even more raw vegetable salads and prevent all sugar. Sugar feeds bacteria and yeast-based infections, and you ought to eliminate processed food items as well as foods saturated in sugar. Use natural low carb sweeteners rather than sugar, such as *stevia, erythritol, xylitol, or chicory root*.

Avoid antibiotic drugs and antibiotic creams when you can, as they are only going to create a temporary fix and result in an overgrowth of candida.

Many doctors prescribe strong antibiotic creams such as **Dalacin V** or strong antifungal drugs such as **Diflucan** because they could be toxic towards the liver, particularly if used repetitively. One harmless treatment for candida may be the usage of vaginal pessaries containing boric acid in a dose of 600mg per pessary, which can be used for two weeks. Another beneficial and harmless treatment would be to douche the vagina having a weak solution of tea tree oil.

The brand called ***Thursday Plantation*** makes a feminine hygiene gel that is blended with warm sterile water (boil water 1st to sterilize it). Mix the gel with the correct amount of water according to the label instructions and fill the douche balloon with this.

Lie within a vacant bath and place the douche nozzle in the vagina and flush the perfect solution is into the vaginal cavity. This can flush out the surplus mucus inside the vagina where the bacteria and candida live.

Tea tree oil works well against bacteria, candida along with other yeasts can prevent them from growing and therefore causing the odor.

The tea tree oil includes a cleansing fresh fragrance, and when the gel solution is blended with the right amount of water, according to the label instructions, there won't exist anything irritating. Some doctors are against douching because they believe that it is not natural or physiological to utilize this practice. I believe it really is much safer than using strong antibiotics and antifungal drugs. Another useful technique is to insert a tablespoon of plain unflavored Greek yogurt into the vagina each day as this can populate the vagina with friendly bacteria that may contend with the unfriendly smelly bacteria. Yogurt keeps the vagina more acidic, which reduces infections. An expert biotic formula may also be swallowed day-by-day to boost the gut flora.

Herpes

Genital herpes is due to infection using the herpes virus (HSV), and it is an extremely common problem that may put a dampener on your own sex life. The original infection of HSV is often very dramatic, with widespread blisters around the vulva. They are painful and frequently connected with fever, pains and aches. Some women experience further recurrent attacks of genital herpes, which varies from monthly to once Atlanta divorce attorneys blue moon.

The antiviral drug called *Acyclovir* works perfectly and reduces symptoms and shortens enough time the blisters can be found. Additional effective antiviral drugs can be found, such as *Valacyclovir* and *Famciclovir,* and the sooner you consider these drugs, the better they work. When you have repeated herpes keep a way to obtain these antiviral drugs in the home. If you're experiencing very frequent recurrent attacks of herpes, you may take Acyclovir every day to suppress the virus, and that means you don't get any blisters or additional symptoms; this also reduces viral shedding from infected areas, thus reducing transmission to your lover. Condoms prevent transmission to your lover. It is critical to prevent excessive stress, as this will likely weaken your disease fighting capability leading to even more frequent attacks, although long-term use of *Acyclovir* can prevent this.

I've found that patients with recurrent herpes benefit greatly by firmly taking a *selenium and zinc supplement*, such as **Selenomune powder**. *Selenium and zinc* are minerals that assist your cell disease fighting capability to fight viruses. I call *selenium* the viral contraceptive pill since it reduces the power of viruses to reproduce and therefore keeps them in a minimal inactive state. In the event that you keep getting frequent attacks of herpes, it is critical to follow an idea to strengthen your complete immune system, which will gradually decrease the frequency and severity of herpes attacks.

Vaginismus

The word *vaginismus* describes the involuntary spasm from the muscles around the vagina when an entry in the vagina is attempted during sex or perhaps a pelvic examination. The effectiveness of the muscular contractions can be quite high so that entry with the vagina is impossible, which could cause extreme discomfort for the person and the girl. The most frequent cause of *vaginismus* is anxiety and fear, perhaps on the unknown, or simply stimulated from the memory of rape or sexual abuse.

Another possible reason behind vaginismus is really a physical abnormality within the pelvic cavity and vagina such as pelvic infection, bladder infection, or endometriosis. These problems could cause pain on attempted entry from the vagina, which can lead to protective muscle spasm. It's essential to visit a specialist gynaecologist for any pelvic exam (when possible) or even a pelvic ultrasound scan at least; these tests will exclude physical factors behind vaginal spasm and pain. Once diagnosed, vaginismus is most beneficially treated by a specialist sex therapist, who could be a health care provider or psychologist; they'll use counseling, relaxation exercises as well as perhaps actually some hypnosis.

Hypnotherapy can be quite effective. It is critical to focus on improving self-confidence. The sex therapist will most likely have to teach you how to employ vaginal dilators to relax and desensitize your vaginal tissues; these work nicely, although a complete cure might take many years. This is something that can't be rushed and should be done at its own pace. Frequent exercises, yoga, and Pilates also may help a whole lot. A magnesium supplement will relax your nervous system as well as your muscles.

Pain in the region of the vulva

Some women experience chronic or recurrent discomfort in the mouth and/or vestibule with the vulva; this tissue is named *vulvodynia*. It's very uncomfortable and could feel just like a dull ache, a burning, stinging feeling, a pressure, rawness, and an itch or a combined mix of each one of these sensations. It is usually connected with unpleasant sexual intercourse.

The reason is usually somewhat mysterious and varies and continues to be deposited to dysfunctional nerve endings within the vulva or nerve injury. The vulva, and especially the part referred to as the vestibule, contains plenty of dense nerve fibers, and if they are dysfunctional, then it's no wonder that severe chronic pain can persist. When the vestibule is touched by a health care provider or possibly a sexual partner, even very lightly, it feels painful. Many sufferers think it is impossible to utilize tampons, and sexual activity may be agonizing or impossible. Often women with vulvodynia haven't enjoyed sex as a result of this pain plus they seek to avoid it.

Just what exactly causes the nerve pain?

There were many theories submit as well as the most logical is chronic inflammation inside the nerve endings and/or in your skin on the vulva; generally, one cannot discover this inflammation on the physical study of the vulva; thus, it is microscopic. Women with vulvodynia will possess chronic inflammation within the bladder wall, which is named interstitial cystitis, which in turn causes unpleasant and frequent urination. When you have *vulvodynia*, it's important to visit a gynaecologist who specializes in this area.

The specialist doctor will eliminate diseases that could masquerade as vulvodynia but require a different treatment. These diseases include skin diseases such as *eczema, lichen planus, lichen sclerosis, contact dermatitis, autoimmune diseases, and infections.* An over-all practitioner may miss or misdiagnose these disorders. The treating vulvodynia will need time and may become very successful if you're persistent and patient. The main thing is usually to lessen the inflammation that's causing the pain inside the nerves and your skin. These strategies work because they're treating the cause, although it might take 6 to a year to understand this inflammation completely in order. Other treatments could be tried like a topical local anaesthetic gel (such as *Xylocaine*) put on the agonizing areas, particularly if you intend to attempt the sexual activity.

Cortisone creams reduce inflammation by suppressing it and will be utilized for flare-ups; however, stay away from daily long-term use. *Castor oil and zinc cream* (utilized for diaper rash) can be quite soothing and protective from the thin skin in the vestibule. When you have a whole lot of anxiety and stress, get one of these strong magnesium supplements such as Magnesium Ultrapotent powder, to calm the central nervous system plus the nerves within the vulva. In highly stressed women who cannot rest, the use of a minimal dose of any tricyclic anti-depressant can greatly dull the pain with least you'll get effective deep sleep.

I emphasize the use of a little dose of your *tricyclic antidepressant* to be utilized initially; you then will not obtain any unwanted effects such as sedation and constipation. These small doses could be made up with a compounding pharmacist.

Urinary tract infections

In a few women, sex aggravates an inclination to urinary tract infections. The urethra is quite close to the opening of the vagina so that it is easy to comprehend how thrusting on the penis could push bacteria up into the urethra or for the urethra to be traumatized and irritated. You might have heard about honeymoon cystitis, which can be an acute bladder infection carrying out a night's passionate sex.

It's a convincing way to ruin your honeymoon! If you're prone to repeat urinary tract infections or interstitial cystitis, endeavor to strengthen your disease fighting capability. This will likely prevent most urinary tract infections, as well as gradually overcome interstitial cystitis. Take extra vitamin C each day within a dose of 1000 to 3000mg.

Prolapse from the pelvic floor and/or vagina

Some women believe that their vagina is too large plus they cannot control the muscles around their vagina. That is common after multiple childbirths, and it produces an inability to contract the vaginal muscles around the penis and frequently reduces sensitivity. In such instances, ask your physician to refer you to definitely a physiotherapist who can educate you on pelvic floor exercises. This often works very well, and you may practise these exercises while driving, washing the laundry, or watching television.

It will provide you with far better control of your bladder as well and frequently overcomes bladder control problems. Such physiotherapists have machines that electrically stimulate the vaginal and pelvic floor muscles, which educate you on which muscles you will need to strengthen. It will always be worth talking to a physiotherapist who specializes on this are. In a few women, the walls in the vagina begin to descend beyond your vaginal opening, and you may experience these bulges at the front end or backward of your vagina.

That is called *prolapse,* of course; if it becomes worse, it could drag down the low to a part of your bladder and rectum. You might feel embarrassed concerning this, and it could hinder bladder and colon control. An excellent gynecologist can simply fix these prolapses via vaginal surgery and tighten the vagina at the same time by detaching the surplus and floppy tissues. You'll be completely new again with a smaller vagina, no prolapse.

Constipation

If you 've constipation, faeces can accumulate inside the rectum, and you'll feel this once the penis pushes backwards within your vagina, which could make it hard for you to relax. To overcome constipation, pelvic floor exercises might help so also can yoga and Pilates. Drink much more water and raise the amount of raw fruit and veggies in your dietary plan. Make use of a *gluten-free fiber* such as Fibertone Powder, and take 2 tablespoons of ground flaxseeds daily.

Poor blood circulation for the vulva

The sexual response and orgasm take a massive amount of blood to flow into the vulva and vaginal arteries in case this will not occur; it'll be much harder to also be lubricated to orgasm. There are factors that may reduce this blood circulation, such as *diabetes, smoking, and high blood pressure.* To boost the blood flow, we can take various natural supplements, and we have to take them regularly.

The main one to take is *magnesium*, and the powder called Magnesium Ultrapotent provides 400mg of highly absorbed magnesium in a single teaspoon. It includes a pleasant flavor, is sweetened with stevia, and works fast, usually within 20 minutes. *Vitamin C helps to enhance the health of the arteries, and I would recommend you take 1000mg daily. Liquid fish oil is of great benefit to boost the blood flow, and I would recommend you purchase an excellent brand and keep it refrigerated.* Take the recommended dose on the label, although if your circulation is quite poor, you might need a higher dose, which is fairly safe to take.

Chapter 8

Treatment Options for Low Libido

There are three different bio-identical sex hormones
- ✓ Progesterone
- ✓ Estrogen
- ✓ Testosterone

Progesterone therapy

Progesterone is a sex hormone that's made by the ovaries during the latter half of the menstrual cycle and in vast amounts by the placenta during pregnancy. Progesterone exerts a calming effect and can promote emotional contentment and stability. The brain has receptors for progesterone, and this is why natural hormones can be so beneficial for emotional disorders. If you find that your mood and/or sex drive is lower during the one to two weeks before your menstrual bleeding commences, then you will probably benefit from natural progesterone. Progesterone deficiency is very common in women today because they often delay pregnancy to later in life and have fewer pregnancies.

Progesterone deficiency can cause unpleasant symptoms such as loss of sex drive, anxiety, irritability, and depression. Progesterone deficiency can also cause physical health problems such as heavy and/or painful menstrual bleeding, endometriosis, fibroids, pelvic congestion, an increased risk of cancer, premenstrual headaches, polycystic ovarian syndrome, and unexplained infertility. The good news is that natural progesterone therapy can often alleviate these symptoms in women of all ages. Thus one would think that natural progesterone is commonly prescribed for these diverse and common problems. In reality, few doctors prescribe natural progesterone because it cannot be patented by drug companies.

Thus, drug companies do not promote natural progesterone or educate doctors about its benefits. It is a pity that this results in much-unneeded suffering.

Natural Progesterone

I recommend only the use of natural progesterone, which has a chemical structure identical to the progesterone produced by the ovaries. Natural progesterone is manufactured within the laboratory through the plant hormone called *diosgenin* within soybeans and sweet potatoes (yams). This is because natural progesterone is identical to the progesterone produced by the ovaries; it is called a bio-identical hormone.

Unfortunately, doctors often prescribe strong synthetic progesterone called **'*progestogens'***, mistakenly believing that they will have the same effect as natural progesterone. This is not true, and synthetic progesterone will usually make most of your symptoms worse and will not help your sex drive. Many of these synthetic progestogens are derived from male (testosterone-like) synthetic hormones, and so may cause side effects such as increased appetite, depression, irritability, low libido, weight gain, fluid retention, acne, greasy skin, and increased cholesterol.

These synthetic progestogen hormones is attached to the natural progesterone receptors found throughout the body and brain, but they cannot switch on all these receptors. Only natural progesterone can turn on ALL the progesterone receptors just as a key turns and releases a lock. So you can understand that synthetic progestogens will not have the same beneficial effect as natural progesterone. Natural progesterone is not as effective if taken by mouth (orally), as it is destroyed by the liver enzymes after its absorption from the intestines.

Therefore, natural progesterone is best administered by routes that bypass the liver such as

- **Creams:** which may be rubbed into the skin (transdermal) or inserted high up into the vagina
- **Vaginal pessaries or suppositories**: Natural progesterone can also be given in the form of *lozenges* known as ***troches***, which are NOT designed to be sucked or chewed or swallowed. Theoretically, the troche is held between the upper gum and the cheek until it is completely absorbed, with the hormone it get being transferred directly into the bloodstream across the mucous lining of the oral cavity. Natural progesterone can also be administered in the form of capsules that contain tiny (micronized) particles of progesterone. Theoretically, these tiny particles of progesterone

are more resistant to breakdown by the enzymes in the gut and the liver so that more progesterone gets into the bloodstream. By giving natural progesterone in these ways, we are aiming to bypass the liver so that the progesterone can be absorbed directly into the circulation and carried for the progesterone receptors on your own cells.

How to work with Natural Progesterone

Generally, natural progesterone therapy is started five days following the end of the menstrual bleeding. The progesterone is then continued daily up to the first day of your menstrual bleeding. Once your bleeding starts the progesterone ought to be stopped. If you find it difficult to judge when to begin using the progesterone, you can start it at the time of ovulation, which is normally 14 days before the expected onset of your menstrual bleeding.

Make sure you stop the progesterone on the first day of your menstrual bleeding, and this way, the progesterone is fitting in with your natural cycle. Each woman is an individual, and trial and error using different dosages, forms, and schedules of progesterone may be required before the symptoms are entirely under control. My personal preference is to administer natural progesterone in the form of a cream, which is rubbed into the skin of the inner upper arms or the inner upper thighs.

You should apply the cream to dry skin after your shower, and if you shower or bathe twice daily, then it may be more effective to apply the cream twice daily after each shower. The cream needs to be rubbed very thoroughly onto the skin so that the entire amount is well absorbed into the skin, with no cream remaining visible or detectable on the skin. The cream can be used once or twice daily, and required doses vary.

The average effective doses are 30mg to 100mg daily. Some doctors are very cynical about the use of creams containing natural progesterone because they do not believe that the progesterone is effectively absorbed through the skin into the bloodstream. In other words, they do not think that clinically effective amounts of progesterone can be achieved in the body by using the creams. However, a study published in the American

Journal of Obstetrics & Gynecology in 1999 found that absorption of progesterone from creams was just as good as absorption of estrogen from patches. They concluded that the application of progesterone cream to the skin appeared to be a safe and effective route of administration.

Progesterone Troches

Natural Progesterone troches are lozenges that are placed between the upper gum and the cheek. They slowly dissolve through the mucous membrane of the cheek along with the progesterone, is absorbed straight into the circulation. Do not suck, chew, or swallow the lozenges. They can be found in a number of flavors. Capsules containing micronized progesterone could be swallowed.

The common dose is 50mg daily; however, the dose may range between 25mg to 200mg regularly. It is given for the 2 weeks before menstrual bleeding. The advantages of the *progesterone troches* are they are convenient to transport around, and just like the progesterone cream, they relieve the symptoms of premenstrual syndrome such as *low libido, mood disorders, insomnia, pelvic congestion, migraines, severe bleeding, menstrual pain, and fatigue.* If doses are excessive, some breakthrough bleeding, drowsiness, and water retention may happen. In a few women, the troche may produce irritation of the gum. In allergy-prone people, the troches could cause allergic-type symptoms such as rashes and swelling.

The progesterone cream is best used in allergy-prone people. If the troches contain sugar, they may increase dental caries. If these side effects occur, then reduce the dosage of hormones in the troche or change to the progesterone cream. Natural progesterone is not a contraceptive and indeed will increase fertility! Natural progesterone does not work if you are taking the oral contraceptive pill. You will need a doctor's prescription for natural progesterone, and it is made up into a cream by a compounding pharmacist in Australia. In the USA, a prescription is not needed, although this may change.

Unwanted effects of Natural Progesterone

Possible unwanted effects consist of some breakthrough bleeding if doses are excessive. Breakthrough bleeding is much more likely to occur when the cream is inserted high up in the vagina. When used vaginally, some vaginal irritation might occur if the bottom with the cream is unsuitable.

In the event, the progesterone cream causes vaginal irritation, get hold of your compounding pharmacist about changing the bottom of the cream. Alternatively, just utilize the cream on your skin from the inner upper arms or inner legs. Excessive doses of progesterone can result in bloating and drowsiness. When you have negative effects, decrease the dose for unwanted effects to disappear. As you can plainly see the mandatory dose may differ a whole lot, as every woman can be a specific, and by tinkering with the dose in the cream, you may steer clear of any unwanted nuisance effects.

How Safe is Natural Progesterone?

Natural progesterone is quite safe and is normally free of unwanted effects. Pure natural progesterone will not cause congenital disabilities or injury to the fetus if you get pregnant and can reduce your likelihood of miscarriage. If you do fall pregnant while taking progesterone, continue steadily to utilize it for the initial 2-3 three months of pregnancy. Notify your physician if you work with progesterone once you fall pregnant.

Synthetic Progesterone

Synthetic progesterone (also called progestogens) can be found, and common brands are *Norethisterone, Norgesterol, and Medroxyprogesterone acetate tablets*. These tablets could be given each day, or for the 2 weeks before menstrual bleeding begins. The dosage varies depending on the make of tablet as well as the medical reason behind which it really is prescribed. These synthetic progestogens have a slightly masculine effect, which might result in putting on weight, pimples, greasy skin, and hair.

Some brands could cause water retention, moodiness, depression, and elevation of cholesterol. They often make depression, as well as other mood disorders much worse. They'll not support your libido and may possess the reverse effect, leading you to be considerably more disinterested in sex!

Estrogen therapy

Natural estrogens may improve libido and sexual response which is particularly true in the below cases;

- Pre-menopausal and post-menopausal women.
- After hysterectomy or after surgical sterilization with tubal clips; in such cases, the ovaries might not work as good after surgery.

Estrogens enhance the condition of the vagina and vulva and also have the following effects;

- Strengthen and thicken the tissues making them better quality - thus you could tolerate longer sex or stronger sex.
- Reduce dryness with the vagina and vulva.
- Increase vaginal secretions.
- Increase vaginal flexibility and stretchiness
- Improve bladder function and reduce bladder infections
- Estrogen can raise the desire to have sex and in addition, makes the breasts and nipples more sensitive to touch. Estrogen keeps the breasts fuller and less droopy.

Types of Natural Estrogen

There are three types of natural estrogen produced by the ovaries and the fat tissue within you; these are referred to as **Estradiol, Estriol, and Estrone**. If you want to have estrogen replacement therapy, it really is desirable to make use of bioidentical estrogens rather than synthetic or animal-derived estrogens such as **Premarin**. Bio-identical estrogens are synthesized inside a laboratory from plant hormones, namely *diosgenin in yams* and *stigmasterol in soybeans*. Bio-identical estrogens can be found in three different forms

- Estradiol = E 2 may be the most potent estrogen
- Estrone = E 1 is of medium strength
- Estriol = E 3 may be the weakest estrogen of all three estrogens.

Estriol

Estriol is the safest of most types of estrogen therapy. Despite the fact that estriol isn't a powerful estrogen, it has been established to work for women with *atrophic vaginitis*. The symptoms of atrophic vaginitis include *vaginal dryness, vaginal burning and irritation, vaginal itching, and unpleasant sexual intercourse*. Unpleasant sexual intercourse is recognized as *dyspareunia* and is often due to low estrogen levels. In most cases, after four weeks of treatment with estriol cream, the symptoms of atrophic vaginitis are relieved.

Other good news is the fact that estriol cream is free from side effects, aside from an exceptionally rare chance for allergy to the bottom found in the cream. Estriol cream also has been found to help prevent urinary tract infections in women with low estrogen levels. Estriol cream may also significantly reduce bladder control problems due to weak pelvic floor muscles, laughing, coughing, and straining. The estriol cream could be inserted into the vagina or rubbed within the vulva, along with the vaginal opening.

Women on natural hormones may begin to behave in a far more provocative way! All three estrogens could be given by means of *creams, troches, tablets, gels, or patches*. These estrogens could be given singly or in mixture; for example something called **Triest** contains all three of the bio-identical estrogens, and **Best** contains estradiol and estriol.

Estrogens could be used cyclically for just two to three weeks on a monthly basis or used each day. It's essential to provide some type of progesterone using the estrogen, and I prefer natural progesterone since it works more effectively and safer. The safest way to manage estrogen can be by using creams or patches as the estrogen is certainly absorbed through your skin into the bloodstream and will not feel the liver; thus we usually do not boost the threat of blood clots.

If estrogen is given via your skin in creams or patches, you won't raise the liver's production of **Sex Hormone Binding Globulin (SHBG),** thus; you may find it sexier! Estrogen creams could be inserted into the vagina or applied to the outside from the vaginal opening (throughout the vulva). In any event this prevents dryness and restores natural lubrication. Only small doses of estrogen are needed, and I mostly use Estriol in a day-by-day dose of 1mg to 2 mg. A doctor's script is necessary for all those three types of estrogen.

Most doctors use branded estrogen creams such as *Ovestin*, that can come with a vaginal applicator to insert the cream high up into the vagina. Ovestin provides the bio-identical estrogen called *Estriol*. Other styles of estrogen such as estrogen tablets or estrogen implants could be used, although they are relatively stronger and, therefore, much more likely to cause unwanted effects such as tender breasts, migraines, leg cramps, water retention and an elevated threat of blood clots.

The estrogen implants are relatively powerful and could cause a rise in menstrual bleeding along with other symptoms of estrogen dominance; thus, they may be best used only in women who've had a hysterectomy. This is because the results in the Women's Health Initiative Study were published in July 2002; all doctors have grown to be aware that long-term estrogen therapy increases the chance of breast cancer. In case the estrogen is normally coupled with synthetic progesterone, this sort of hormone therapy becomes a lot more risky to work with long-term, with an elevated threat of blood clots and strokes.

Thus it isn't wise to make use of strong types of estrogen therapy for quite some time, and this implies that estrogen implants are only ideal for short term employ. This applies for only one year. Excessive doses or the stronger types of estrogen are best avoided because they can result in symptoms of estrogen dominance.

Estrogen dominance symptoms can include

- Breast pain and lumpiness
- Water retention
- Gallstones
- Heavy or painful menstrual bleeding
- Increased size of fibroids
- Migraines
- Aching legs and leg cramps
- Blood clots
- Putting on weight inside the hips and thighs.

If these unwanted effects occur, you'll need your physician to lessen the dosage of estrogen or change to the weakest type of estrogen that is *estriol*. I've found that small doses of the estriol cream usually do not produce any unwanted effects and this is usually my preferred treatment, specifically for older women or for long-term work. Both natural progesterone and estrogens will certainly reduce insomnia and hot flushes.

Testosterone therapy

Testosterone is created from cholesterol within the ovaries, adrenal glands, and fat tissues. Testosterone can be a healthy hormone in both sexes, so when it involves libido; it could end up being called the hormone of desire. It works to promote sexual desire in our brain, and our genital organs and these regions of the body contain testosterone receptors. Testosterone receptors are located in the cells of the nipples, the clitoris, and vagina. Some women have surprisingly low degrees of testosterone while others produce an excessive amount. Your degree of testosterone is easily and accurately measured, having a blood test. It's important to gauge the degrees of both total testosterone and free testosterone, which are circulating inside your blood.

The test for total testosterone measures the absolute amount of testosterone within your blood, like the amount that's bound to the protein *Sex Hormone Binding Globulin (SHBG)*. **SHBG** functions just like a transport vehicle to transport the testosterone around your bloodstream towards the organs of your body that require it. Once the testosterone is broken from the SHBG it becomes free and is also thus in a position to act on your cells. It is simply the free testosterone that is active on your cells, and therefore, it's the kind of testosterone that promotes libido.

The data below demonstrate the quantity of total testosterone in the blood that's considered normal.

- **Women Total testosterone**: 30 - 95ng/dL (nanograms per deciliter).
- **Men Total testosterone**: 300 to at least 1,200ng/dL (nanograms per deciliter).

In case a male's testosterone levels drop below 500, their libido will certainly reduce, often dramatically. In women, you can see that these testosterone levels are lower than in men, and the standard range is a lot narrower. This means that your body is going to be sensitive to relatively small changes in your blood testosterone level. For instance, a reduction or a rise by

20ng/dl could make a significant difference for your sexuality.

Low degrees of testosterone could cause the next symptoms
- Low libido
- Reduced capability to orgasm
- A decrease in how big is your clitoris
- A decrease in the sensitivity of your respective clitoris
- A decrease in sexual fantasies
- Muscle pains and aches or muscle weakness
- Backache and chest wall pain
- Reduction of/or lack of pubic and armpit (axillary) hair

Low degrees of testosterone could be caused by:
- Hysterectomy with removal of the ovaries; in a few women, even if the ovaries are left set up throughout a hysterectomy (surgery on the uterus), we discover that the sex hormone levels drop to surprisingly low levels rather than recover.

- Adrenal gland exhaustion or adrenal gland failure; thus, it's important to get healthy adrenal gland function to supplement your production of testosterone.
- The oral contraceptive pill, which increases SHBG, which binds the testosterone.
- Postnatal depression.
- The pre-menopausal years if the ovaries are aging and gradually producing less testosterone as well as other sex hormones.
- The post-menopausal years once the ovaries shrink and are inactive, although smaller amounts of testosterone continue being created from the ovaries also a long time after menopause, but also for many women it is nowhere near enough to allow them to look sexually alive.

Surprisingly low degrees of testosterone is additionally observed in women with a minimal bodyweight and a minimal muscle mass. The body type can influence the quantity of testosterone that you produce.

Women who are overweight and carry the majority of their unwanted weight within the chest muscles and abdomen frequently have excess degrees of testosterone and could have an increased libido as a result of this. This physique is named the *apple shape*.

If an overweight, thin-shaped woman consumes high levels of carbohydrate foods, especially sugar, this may lead to an elevated production of testosterone. If an thin-shaped woman consumes more protein, this can result in lower degrees of testosterone. Thus our diet makes a difference in our hormones.

Ways of using Testosterone

The ultimate way to balance the testosterone levels in a female has been a cream containing natural bio-identical testosterone. This testosterone is manufactured within a laboratory using plant hormones such as diosgenin, as the starting material. Bio-identical hormones own the precise shape and structure as your own body's naturally produced hormones.

Bio-identical hormones have already been popularized with the media and celebrities, and I get that many women know they are safer than synthetic hormones. Previously, if a female needed testosterone replacement she'd usually be prescribed an artificial kind such as **methyltestosterone** by means of tablets or injections. *Methyltestosterone* includes a different chemical structure to your body's own naturally produced testosterone and is a lot more potent than bio-identical testosterone. *Methyltestosterone* was administered in tablet form and, as a result of this, was immediately processed from the liver after it had been absorbed in the gut; thus the liver broke the majority of it down before it would enter the bloodstream. As a result of this, high doses of *methyltestosterone* were needed and thus unwanted effects such as masculinization and putting on weight were more prevalent.

Therefore many women had been turned off using any male hormones to promote their sexual drive. If we use testosterone creams, we can bypass the liver as the testosterone is absorbed via your skin into the blood circulation and is carried around your body to the cells that require it. All of this happens prior to the liver can break it down. That is much safer, as only minimal doses of testosterone become effective in this manner. The reduced doses found in the cream act like the levels of testosterone made by your ovaries and adrenal glands, and therefore they don't produce big changes in your blood testosterone levels. We can easily adjust or titrate the dose of the testosterone you will need without any unwanted effects being produced.

One effect we do want to see, however, is a boost in your libido and sexual pleasure. I find that the use of a cream containing testosterone allows the dose of testosterone to be easily measured and adjusted.

For instance, if we get the compounding pharmacy to produce a testosterone cream containing 5mg of testosterone per gram of cream, we can measure amounts from 1/10th (.10) of a gram to at least 1 gram utilizing a 1ml syringe or a 1 gram spoon. One gram is the same as a 1ml level of the cream. If we started with 1 ml (1gram) of the cream, we are receiving 5 mg of testosterone, and we can try this for several weeks to see if your libido improves. If you're concerned about potential unwanted effects, focus on 1/10th (.10) of a gram. It is possible to adjust the dose down or up dependant on your response.

The concentration of the testosterone in the cream may also be varied by the prescribing doctor and the compounding dispensing pharmacist, so you may choose to get one of these lower strength creams of 1mg of testosterone per gram of cream for instance. I've found that was to use the testosterone cream is on the vulva and ensure you get some of the clitorides. Some women just apply it to the clitoris, which is effective for them. That's where the testosterone must work to keep your clitoris a standard size also to promote sensitivity of the clitoris and lips of the vulva. The body may also absorb a number of the testosterone from the vulva into the bloodstream, which means this should boost your blood degrees of testosterone into the normal healthy range.

After beginning testosterone cream, you need to spot the difference within 14 days. The cream can be used each day or every second-day dependant on your taste and is certainly rubbed onto the clitoris and vulva. Apply the cream after your shower or very last thing during the night and rub it on well; you don't want to waste it, it is expensive. Usually, do not apply just before sex, or your partner will be getting some of your testosterone! Bio-identical testosterone can be micronized and put in a capsule for swallowing.

The term micronized means very fine particles that are theoretically better absorbed from a capsule. However, the micronized testosterone, once absorbed from the gut, passes straight to the liver, and the liver can easily break it down because it is a natural hormone. Natural hormones are much easier for the liver to break down than synthetic hormones. I prefer to use testosterone creams, and I generally do not prescribe testosterone capsules because of its liver effect. Testosterone can be given in the form of troches, which are *lozenges* designed to be placed between the gum and the cheek. The troche needs to be kept in that position for around 20 minutes to allow the hormones to be absorbed across the mucus lining of the cheek directly into the blood circulation. I don't prescribe troches very much because it is unavoidable that some of the hormones in the troche will be swallowed and thus go through the liver.

This means that higher doses of hormones must be used in the troches compared to the creams. However, some women prefer the troches and find them effective. Some women are very sensitive to testosterone and will get side effects if they use too much.

Side effects of excess testosterone include;
- Increase in facial hair,
- Scalp hair loss especially in the frontal and temporal areas of the scalp,
- Acne and pimples,
- Increased aggression in mood and also in the bedroom!

In this case, your partner may come to see your doctor, also asking for help to have his testosterone levels increased! Some doctors do not understand the art and science of balancing a woman's hormones to make her feel just right when it comes to her sexuality. Many peri-menopausal and post-menopausal women struggle to restore their hormonal balance and libido because they are given the wrong doses and types of hormones.

They need to feel helpless when faced with a woman who has a hormonal mess and wants her libido back -- if not! That is why you need to educate yourself, which means you can let the doctor know what you require or else seek the services of a doctor who specializes in ***bio-identical sex hormones.***

Just as women need to be assertive in the bedroom, they need to be assertive with their doctors, and you can do it in a non-confrontational way and even suggest to the doctor what you would like in your cream. Some women take the hormone DHEA (spelled ***dehydroepiandrosterone***) because they think it works the same as testosterone. They also think that it can get turned into testosterone and estrogen in their ovaries. This not true, as once your ovaries have stopped making hormones, they cannot use any raw material type hormones. **DHEA** acts in your body like a weaker form of testosterone, but it does not have the libido enhancing effects of real testosterone.

I use **DHEA** in women with poor adrenal gland function and chronic fatigue, and it is helpful for these problems. I have had patients addicted to testosterone because it makes them feel like a superwoman! One particular patient, who is in her 50s, gets her local doctor to give her testosterone injections every month, and these injections contain a high dose. She does have some extra facial and body hair and a slightly deep voice, but she does not care! If she does not get her testosterone shots, she feels 200 years old and has awful fatigue, depression, and muscle and bone pain. She does not use testosterone primarily for sex drive, but she uses it for her wellbeing.

Another patient of mine had suffered from a chronic backache and chest wall pain for 20 years. After 6 weeks on testosterone replacement, she was pain-free and no longer needed to take pain killers. Wow, that's impressive!

Aside from its sexual enhancing effects, testosterone has other results and may;
- Boost energy

- Reduce depression
- Reduce muscle and bone pain
- Increase bone relative density
- Increase muscle bulk and muscle strength,

Note: *Do not overdose testosterone, or you may change from superwoman into a superman!*

Is Testosterone Safe?

Generally speaking, low doses of bio-identical testosterone are very safe. This logical, as we are only using treatments that keep the blood levels of testosterone in the normal or physiological range. This is what your ovaries and adrenal glands would do if they were working properly. With age, however, their hormonal output diminishes, and we begin to suffer the symptoms of testosterone deficiency.

Oral synthetic testosterone is not as safe as the low doses of natural testosterone used in the creams. Large doses of synthetic testosterone may cause an increase in cholesterol levels. If you take long term hormones, you need your regular blood checks of cholesterol levels and liver function in addition to checking your levels of testosterone and other hormones. If the testosterone level is too high, we simply reduce the dose, which is easy to do with cream.

You will not become masculinized if small doses of testosterone are used. There are few long term studies on the use of testosterone, but I believe it is normally very safe, and I have never seen it cause any serious side effects or cancer.

Aside from its sexual enhancing effects, testosterone has other results, they are
- Boost energy
- Reduce depression
- Reduce muscle and bone pain
- Increase bone relative density
- Increase muscle bulk and muscle strength

But we usually do not need to overdose on testosterone, or we might change from superwoman into superman!

Chapter 9
Enhancing Sexual Drive in Men
Muscle Mass Building and Testosterone Enhancing

One thing you need to understand about having even more testosterone is you'll want to eat the proper foods. This implies you must begin to introduce healthy fat in what you eat, regardless of how strange that sounds. Yes, it's true. The good sort of fat is actually best for your body. This is because something is oily doesn't mean it'll do nothing befitting the body, and you need to prevent it altogether.

This is due to the first days of the Pro-testosterone Diet, and the forming of testosterone or water-soluble molecules that come from essential fatty acids, and they are made by the liver when your body enters the state of carbohydrate restriction, which prompts it to turn glucose into energy carefully. Two of the given testosterone above will be the ones converted into vigor that the mind and heart may use. At the same time, acetone simply becomes a degradation from acetoacetic acid.

They are transported from the liver completely to various other tissues in the torso and therefore are found in most physiologic conditions. Actually, the mind gets 25% of its energy from testosterone, and may possibly produce Omega-3 essential fatty acids that will avoid the body from deteriorating or aging fast.

Using the discovery of the testosterone, Woodyatt, regarding his colleague Mynie Peterman, thought the formulation of a high-fat, low-carb diet would be substantial for those who desire to build up muscle, strengthen their bodies, obtain ideal weight, and keep themselves safe from epilepsy and diabetes because it produces a whole lot of testosterone.

Peterman then formulated the first **Pro-testosterone Diet**, which involves a gram of protein per kilogram of the child's body weight. Which means that he'd gain the majority of his calorie consumption, and 10 to 15% from carbohydrates. Nowadays, it's said which you can use at least 40% fat, 40% protein, and 20% carbohydrates to assist you to gain muscles and ensure that your testosterone levels increase.

What to Eat

Bacon Burgers.

Again, some salt and protein can do you a whole lot of great. Bacon burgers can help you acquire that spare boost of energy, and they're wonderful to consume during snack time or lunch, too. You can amp it up with the addition of cauliflower rice for the mixture of your meat, or some garlic to provide it that surplus kick.

Chocolate Peanut Butter Shake.

Peanut Butter is really among the healthiest types of fats available. With the ability to satisfy your sweet tooth without causing you to fear that you'll have diabetes roughly since it doesn't have a whole lot of carbohydrates. Add cottage cheese to the mix, and you'll experience a drink you could pair together with your meals again! It's also better to drink this before and after a good work out.

Nut-Crusted Salmon.

It's not really a secret that salmon is among the best proteins not to say fish, because they have Omega-3 essential fatty acids, as well as proteins that the body must live. It's easy to get ready and consume what you would like if you wish to gain more muscle and testosterone.

Short Ribs.

Produce Cajun or Asian-style ones, and surely, you'd have something amazing to consume for lunch. Apart from being truly a high-fat dish, these ribs will also be tender and delicious. It's grilled, has that pickled think, which is something you'd wish to devour immediately.

Grilled Salmon.

Salmon is filled up with Omega-3 essential fatty acids and the proper amount of protein, particularly when cooked skin side down on a grill. Allow smoke cook the fish's top portion so you'd get yourself a large amount of meat.

No-Bun Burgers.

By firmly taking away the buns, you can add much healthier fats towards the burgers, which might contain avocados, bacon, cheese, eggs, or peanut butter. In this manner, you get yourself a large number of ketones with just one single bite-and never have to do with carbohydrate-filled buns!

Roasted Chicken.

This comfort food has a number of the healthiest fats, mainly when baked at 425 degrees or when cooked ten minutes per round!

Slow-Cooker Stew.

Slow-cooked meals are essential in the Protestosterone Diet since it permits you to eat sometimes the toughest meats with no trouble! You get the proper fat content you could turn that into energy very quickly.

Steak and Eggs.

This may be ideal for breakfast or once you feel just like it, particularly if it's sirloin. You can also cook the eggs whichever way you want.

Chapter 10

Herbs For Better Sex

Ginseng, "The King of Most Herbs"

This herb may be the most revered herb in China, Korea, and Japan. They revere it because of its tonifying and anti-aging houses. Most Chinese and Koreans take it for energy throughout the day or if they start to get older to improve their entire body. Legend has it that this famous Chinese monarch Qin Shi Huang regularly ate ginseng, hoping to gain eternal life. King Yeongin lived to become 83, and he also made ginseng a normal part of his diet. Many Emperors of China used ginseng to stay virile as well as for optimum health insurance, and the majority of us need the same results. This sexy root, which appears like a vintage man, is filled with energetic powers that benefit the complete body. Ginseng can be a potent strength tonic and can keep you awake and alert for several hours.

This herb will help you stay also focused to keep your brain alert. What's incredible is the fact that it doesn't simply offer you a boost of vigor, but it additionally supports depression, raised cholesterol, and diminishing libido. In Korea and China, women and men take it each morning when they start to get older so that they don't drop their stamina and vitality. This sexy tonic also really helps to offset general weakness in the muscles, lungs, as well as the male's sexy appendage, so you and your spouse both can possess the strength to go forever or as long as you like, both finishing with smiles on your faces. P.S.

That is **Siberian, Panax, or Korean Ginseng** - not **American ginseng**. The *American species* can be used for insomnia and nourishing the Yin of your body, not the Yang. *Panax or Korean Ginseng* can be bought raw, in pill form, capsules, tea, or tinctures. Additionally, it is one of many ingredients in lots of those energy beverages available on the market, however it isn't the ginseng that hurts your adrenals. It's the sugar and caffeine that in addition they enhance the mix. Having a good cup of ginseng tea won't offer you a nervous buzz that may later make you crash. Ginseng will provide you with a nice feel of vigor and alertness for your day with no jitters. In

China, additionally, it is called the *"wrinkle eraser,"* because this herb can provide you strength and support to erase your wrinkles.

He Shou Wu- Fo-Ti, "Youthful Tonic"

"An attractive weapon against aging." This sexy root and vine may fight to age, increase your vigor, and fortify your bones while maintaining your hair together with your mind healthy and shiny. In addition, it allows you to keep your natural color longer among colorings. A Chinese woman begins drinking this tea when she sees a grey hair. The name **He Shou Wu means**, ***"Mr. He that has beautiful black hair"*** as the legend is the fact Mr. He was an extremely old, grouchy man who lived by himself out in the woods. He was also a stingy man who didn't desire to cover tea, so when he saw this vine growing outside his house, he started cutting it and brewing it like a tea, plus the results were amazing.

His hair turned black again, his wrinkles disappeared, and he had so much strength that he could marry a girl within the village, and he lived long enough to possess many children. Fo-Ti may be the Western name because of this herb, and Western medicine has discovered that it is an "adaptogen." Adaptogens certainly is a super-elite, sexy band of herbs. They have got only found out 18 of the sexy herbs that provide your body what it is missing if you need vigor, it offers you strength; if you don't sleep, it can help you to rest. This herb may also enable you to remember things since it helps to rejuvenate brain cells. The other excellent quality of adaptogens is that they help the body to cope with stress. They stop your adrenal glands from producing cortisol that is yucky hormone that goes crazy whenever we are in constant stress and produces that stomach fat that people can't remove easily. Stress is hard on your body, and after being under constant stress for an extended period of your time, you may burn up your adrenals and cause havoc to your wellbeing.

This sexy herb helps to nourish your adrenals so they obtain second wind, although it also offers you a Zen Master feeling of calmness along with the vigor that may help you make it through the existing crisis. I like this herb since it gives you a good zing of strength, and that means you can jump tall buildings, become Buddha in stressful situations, and also have a definite mind to juggle those balls you might have up in the environment while hair is usually smoking hot. "Aging isn't dropped youth but a fresh stage of opportunity and strength."

Ashwagandha, "Indian Ginseng"

This herb is quite popular in Ayurvedic medicine since it has such wonderful healing properties. Ashwagandha is among the special 18 adaptogens here on earth, so it can provide you vigour. It can help with anxiety while at exactly the same time cutting your cortisol amounts. It also includes a positive influence on your irritable mood and stops your brain from racing to get an excellent night's sleep. Ashwagandha also supports infertility in men and women and will assist you to with minimal libido. Imagine being in an extremely sound mood, having plenty of strength, and having the ability to leave all of your concerns behind you.

You could have sexy nighttime with your honey bunny of preference; the icing within the cake because of this herb is the fact that after your sexy night, you'll be able to enjoy an excellent night's sleep. Out of this moment, you won't need to be worried about being exhausted rather than wanting to become bothered when you are feeling frisky and prepared to fun because you took several drops of the herbal tincture. *Ashwagandha* can be purchased online or at any health grocery. It is bought from capsules or being a tincture. That is among the herbs within the majority of your adrenal tonics. I consider an adrenal tonic every day, and so I understand this sexy herb in my blood system each day. Happiness is only the right health insurance and poor memory.

Guarana, "Sexier when Compared to a Cup of Joe"

This sexy plant is from Venezuela and Brazil, and it packs more punch when compared to a cup of espresso. These little seeds have double the quantity of caffeine than coffee. Guarana has 4.5 grams of caffeine, while coffee has 2.2. This business can help you to get moving in the morning and may put a higher voltage spring within your step. Unless you just like the bitter taste of coffee, nevertheless, you enjoy that jolt of energy that only caffeine can provide you, you then should consider guarana. These sexy seeds are capable of supercharging your time, get your brain to focus, also to keep you sharp and alert.

Guarana will be a sound decision on days you need to have a big exam, execute a presentation, or you must sit through a boring class or meeting. As the others in the area are yawning or are experiencing trouble concentrating, you can ace the exam or presentation and feel just like an attractive winner if you are done. There is nothing more "unsexy" when compared to a foggy brain that has no focus or direction. Wittiness and an instant intellect are sexy tools that work wonders at every age. Maintaining your mind clear and sharp into later years will benefit everyone around you as well as contribute to your current health.

Guarana, also, has been utilized for weight reduction due to the saponins inside the plant. They help burn pesky body fat in the torso. For anybody sensitive to caffeine due to high blood pressure or additional issues, be mindful when purchasing an innocuous energy drink. If you're a tired, sexy one and you must do a presentation or have a meeting to visit and whatever you can consider is usually your pillow, you might like to have some guarana capsules to assist you to perform at your very best. They can be purchased online, or your neighborhood health grocery most likely carries it. Follow the directions for the bottle, and do not take it each day since it will degrade your adrenals. It is for special occasions.

Creatine, "Muscle Powder"

If you want, you could have more vigor and muscle tissue because you are feeling that you will be looking weak as well as your muscle tone is diminishing, you might like to put this powder for your protein drink or green drink each day and you'll build up muscle mass. This powder is quite favored by the weightlifters because they understand that if they require it, they can do more reps, or they can lift heavier weights to create bigger and stronger muscles. Women also have to train strength because we begin to appear flabby and doughy if we don't lift or if we just concentrate exclusively on cardio exercises.

I like aerobics, yoga, and tai chi exercises, but to be sure we've strength, tone, and definition, we should incorporate lifting weights at least 2-3 times each day. If you'd like bigger muscles, then add this powder in your morning drink. The first week which you begin incorporating creatine for your morning regular you will put on weight, but it is going to be drinking water weight before muscles begin to release water and begin building muscle, so just relax, keep training, and you'll commence noticing those beautiful, defined legs and arms as they initiate appearing.

Then placed on those short or sleeveless shirts and begin strutting your stuff. This super supplement isn't just for weight lifters anymore. The elderly are beginning to bring it to greatly help with being less creaky also to have significantly more mobility. Remember, it is only ideal for those sexy seniors who are already performing exercise but are feeling some stiffness and tightness within their bodies. They, too, can do more reps or begin to lift heavier weights. In addition, it helps us to build up muscle mass whenever we start to get older because we lose our muscle tissue as we age. If you're a senior, you ought to be weight lifting 2-3 times weekly and taking creatine powder to be sure you retain your sexy muscles also to preserve you from looking buff.

They also have discovered that creatine helps alleviate depression for individuals who don't respond good to anti-depressants or do not wish to be on medication. Imagine being over 60 and that you will be nonetheless active, flexible, and happy. Given that it is sexy!

If you are in your 60s or above, you are active and need to stay this way; then, you would want to put 5 grams of *Creatine* in your juice each day. Make sure it's pure Creatine Monohydrate when you get it, and drink it quickly after putting it in liquid since it starts wearing down within seconds.

Astragalus, "The Fantastic Body Lifter"

This is an excellent herb for securing the skin in the neck and the one's pesky droopy eyelids. Additionally, it is good for accumulating the *Qi (strength of your body)* so that it gives you vigor. Since it is usually working from The within out, it accumulates your disease fighting capability, so you have more strength, tighter, and lifted skin while at precisely the same time it is producing your disease fighting capability strong with sexy, little white cells playing around keeping you healthy and attractive.

Astragalus *"the fantastic lifter"* means additionally, it may lift saggy skin from your legs and elbows on your body.

Furthermore, it may support women who experience prolapse with the uterus. The only path to place it backward when surgery is done in your 20's. If it has fallen and the physician doesn't want to execute surgery, you might like to get some good *astragalus* or proceed to see your neighborhood acupuncturist because acupuncture might help, and she can mix the astragalus with other herbs to make it stronger. It could be purchased by means of raw, capsules, powder, or tincture online or at your Chinese neighborhood store or health grocery. If you choose the dried kind, it could be put into any soups; just ensure that you rinse and soak it before adding it in the soup because they sometimes spray it with sulfur to preserve it longer.